FOR EVERY PARENT QUESTIONING
WHETHER YOU'RE DOING IT RIGHT.
YOU'VE GOT THIS.

CONTENTS

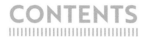

ESSENTIAL
PREGNANCY

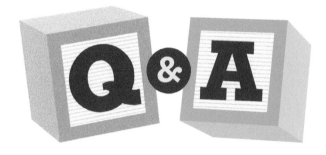

EXPERT ANSWERS and ADVICE
for Every Stage of Your Pregnancy
and Postpartum Journey

BRYN HUNTPALMER
with Dr. Emiliano Chavira, MD, MPH, FACOG
Lindsey Meehleis, LM, CPM
Courtney Butts, LMSW

ROCKRIDGE
PRESS

Interior & Cover Designer: Tricia Jang
Art Producer: Megan Baggott
Editor: Ada Fung
Production Editor: Matt Burnett
Author photo: Heather Gallagher

ISBN: Print 978-1-64611-353-8 | eBook 978-1-64611-354-5

R0

CHAPTER THREE

PHYSICAL AND EMOTIONAL SYMPTOMS 35

CHAPTER FOUR

COMMON ILLNESSES AND AILMENTS 51

CHAPTER FIVE

FOOD AND NUTRITION 59

CHAPTER SIX

ENVIRONMENT, LIFESTYLE, AND SELF-CARE 67

CHAPTER SEVEN

SEX AND EXERCISE 79

CHAPTER EIGHT

WORK AND TAKING LEAVE 85

CHAPTER NINE

PREPARING FOR BABY 91

CHAPTER TEN

LABOR AND CHILDBIRTH 101

CHAPTER ELEVEN

POSTPARTUM CARE 131

CHAPTER TWELVE

FEEDING AND CARING FOR YOUR NEWBORN 149

PREGNANCY AND LABOR COMPLICATIONS 167

CHAPTER FOURTEEN
PREGNANCY LOSS 191

MEET THE PREGNANCY AND POSTPARTUM EXPERTS

DR. EMILIANO CHAVIRA, MD, MPH, FACOG

Dr. Chavira is board certified in Obstetrics & Gynecology with a subspecialty certification in Maternal-Fetal Medicine. He completed both his OB/GYN residency training and his fellowship in Maternal-Fetal Medicine at LAC+USC Medical Center in Los Angeles, California. In his years as a specialist working in tertiary referral centers, he has cared for some very complicated and high-risk pregnancies, dealing with both maternal medical issues and complex fetal problems. He currently serves as Chair of the Women's & Children's Services Department at Martin Luther King Jr. Community Hospital, and as Medical Director for the Del Mar Birth Center, both in the greater Los Angeles area. His passion is to provide objective and caring guidance to his patients with the aim of instilling knowledge, understanding, empowerment, and hope in difficult circumstances. In addition to caring for complicated pregnancies, he also has an interest in ethical dilemmas in modern obstetric care, particularly as related to vaginal breech birth, multiple gestations, and vaginal birth after cesarean (VBAC).

LINDSEY MEEHLEIS, LM, CPM

Lindsey Meehleis is a mum, midwife, and mentor. She graduated from Nizhoni Institute of Midwifery, the only state-accredited midwifery school in California, at the head of her class. Since 2004, she has served thousands of childbearing women and their families, attending births and running a lactation clinic at a local hospital. Lindsey is a midwifery educator, serving as a mentor and trainer for other midwives. She is also a doula, yoga teacher, lactation consultant, Reiki master, Emergency Medical Technician, Water Safety Advocate, and avid user of and educator regarding essential oils since 2006. Her passion lies in empowering women to find their voices and power not only in birth but also in all areas of health and wellness. You can find her on Instagram (@lindseymeehleis), where she shares birth stories and makes it her mission to normalize pregnancy, labor, and childbirth.

COURTNEY BUTTS, LMSW

Courtney is a Licensed Master Social Worker (LMSW), adjunct professor, and certified BEST Doula in Dallas, Texas. She has a Bachelor of Science in Psychology and a Master of Science in Social Work. Specializing in perinatal mental health, intimate-partner violence, and sexual trauma, Courtney became interested in birth work after the birth of her son. Birth work has allowed Courtney to bring together two things she is passionate about: working with trauma survivors and all things pregnancy and postpartum. As a mental health professional, her goal is to provide a safe and compassionate space for individuals and couples to gain a deeper understanding of how their life experiences influence healing and success moving forward.

INTRODUCTION
IIIIIIIIIIIIIIIIIIIIIIIIIIIIIIIIIIIIIIIIIIIIIIII

Learning you're pregnant comes with excitement, but it can also be a time of uncertainty. If this is your first pregnancy, everything about growing a tiny human is new, and you'll likely have questions along the way. Your own concerns are probably amplified by the constant stream of advice and personal anecdotes you're getting from family, friends, and perfect strangers!

When I was pregnant with my first baby, I was obsessed with reading everything I could find on how to have the healthiest pregnancy and birth. Even with all of the reading, questions still came up. I know I'm not alone in turning to Internet searches or the never-ending dark hole of pregnancy forums for answers. I found conflicting information and didn't know which pieces of advice to trust. I didn't want to bother my midwife with every question that came up, so I waited until my checkups to ask my long list of burning questions. I often wished I had my care provider on hand to address the little concerns in between appointments—thus the inspiration for this book!

I rounded up a team of experts—an OBGYN, a midwife, and a therapist specializing in maternal mental health—to help address expecting parents' most frequently asked questions. I also wanted to include real stories from parents in the trenches. I surveyed listeners of *The Birth Hour* and asked them to weigh in on the topics covered in the book. Each chapter opens with an anecdote from someone who has been right where you are. Reading these, you'll quickly realize how many different versions of normal there are when it comes to having a baby!

To make it easier for you to navigate, I've organized this book into topic-based chapters, covering everything from the dos and don'ts of pregnancy to preparing for childbirth to navigating parental leave and postpartum recovery. My hope is that the Q&A format will help you quickly and easily find trustworthy answers to your most pressing pregnancy, labor, and postpartum questions. In other words, I want to help keep you away from those forums and Internet searches as much as possible!

HOW TO USE THIS BOOK

The format of this book is set up for you to search for the answers to your questions as they arise rather than reading a bunch of information that isn't relevant to you and your pregnancy. In writing this book, we intended for you to skip around rather than read the book cover to cover. Since the chapters are topic-based, you should be able to find the information you need quickly, and you can also reference the detailed Table of Contents (page vi), where each question is listed as well.

While the book is mainly focused on the most commonly asked questions, it does cover pregnancy and postpartum complications that may or may not apply to you. You might want to avoid reading those sections unless the need arises so that you aren't adding any unnecessary stress during your pregnancy.

WHEN TO SEEK MEDICAL HELP

Pregnancy can be one of the most wonderful and memorable periods of your life. At the same time, there will inevitably be many questions and worries along the way. This guide will serve as a reliable starting point to address some of those questions. While it was written by a team of pregnancy experts, this book is not a replacement for professional advice from your care provider.

Please use it as a general advice book to help ease anxieties and fears about your pregnancy, labor, and the postpartum period, but always seek medical help if you have any questions or concerns. You should definitely seek evaluation as soon as you discover you're pregnant to see how far along you are and to establish care. Contact your care provider immediately if you experience excessive vomiting, difficulty breathing, severe abdominal pain, severe back pain, vaginal bleeding, persistent headaches or blurred vision, painful swelling, signs of early labor, or decline in baby's movements or if any other concerns arise, especially for any symptom that occurs suddenly or is severe in nature.

For the most part, this book is written for the majority of pregnancies, so if you have preexisting conditions that can complicate pregnancy, some of the advice in this book may not apply to you; consult with your provider for care tailored to your situation.

Know that people call their care providers *all* the time and you aren't going to bother anyone by calling. Most doctors' offices and insurance providers have a 24/7 nurse line to address any concerns that arise, and most midwives would much rather you call or text them with a question than stress over it for a few weeks until your next appointment. It's always better to err on the side of caution and have that extra layer of reassurance!

"You think you know what you'll be like when you are hormonal. Then all of a sudden your sweet husband is driving you up a wall and a vacuum commercial is making you cry. Pregnancy is a very weird time."

—Allē Sanchez

A Quick Guide to the Four Trimesters

Bryn Huntpalmer

◇◇◇◇◇◇◇◇◇◇◇◇◇◇◇◇◇◇◇◇◇◇◇◇◇

This chapter provides an overview of what you can expect at each stage of pregnancy, or trimester, as well as the first three months of baby's life, often called the "fourth trimester." We will go over baby's development, key appointments and testing, and symptoms you may experience. In addition, you'll find some suggestions for ways to take care of yourself and some items to check off your to-do list. Keep in mind that not all appointments and symptoms will apply to everyone, or they may happen on a different timeline. If you ever have any concerns, whether or not they're covered in this book, please consult with your doctor or midwife.

Overview

Your hormones are shifting, so the first trimester often includes the most well-known pregnancy symptoms (e.g., sore breasts, exhaustion, and nausea). But it's also normal not to experience any symptoms in the early days. Now is the time to decide on the type of care provider you want and where you want to give birth, as these are often the most important decisions in determining the type of birth you will have.

Baby Development

Baby develops from an embryo to a fetus, and by the end of the first trimester, the fetus looks like a baby on ultrasound, and all of its major organs are formed and functioning.

Key Appointments and Tests

- Around week 8: First doctor's appointment and possible dating ultrasound (see page 22).
- Around week 10: Decide whether you want genetic testing and schedule it (see page 27).
- Your doctor or midwife will order blood work and collect a urine sample to establish a baseline.
- Around week 12: Second prenatal appointment

Potential Physical and Emotional Symptoms

- Sore breasts
- Mild cramping
- Exhaustion
- Frequent urination
- Increase in vaginal discharge
- Constipation
- Mood swings or mixed feelings about becoming a parent

Food and Nutrition

- If you're too nauseated to keep much food down, don't stress. Keep taking your prenatal vitamin and know that nausea typically eases up in the second trimester.
- Once your appetite returns, focus on iron-rich foods and getting plenty of protein.
- Cut out alcohol.

Lifestyle and Self-Care

- Stop smoking and avoid secondhand smoke.
- Walk daily as you feel up to it.
- Sleep as much as possible.
- Start a journal or mindfulness practice.
- Avoid job duties that involve hazardous fumes, chemicals, or radiation.

To-Do List

- Interview care providers and make your first appointments.
- Explore your options around childbirth.
- Call your insurance company and get out-of-pocket estimates for your pregnancy and birth.

Signs to Seek Medical Advice

- Excessive vomiting
- Severe abdominal pain
- Vaginal bleeding
- If any other concerns arise

Overview

For many pregnant people this is considered the honeymoon trimester because your hormones are leveling out, helping ease pregnancy symptoms, but your belly isn't so big yet that you can't tie your own shoes. You'll have some big appointments this month, including the anatomy scan, during which you can learn your baby's sex if you want. Enjoy this time and plan fun things to do, but I also recommend using these weeks to get things on your "preparing for baby" to-do list done.

Baby Development

- Baby's lungs, heart, and other systems are functioning, and baby can survive outside the womb (with medical help) starting around week 24.
- Baby starts to hear sounds, and its eyes open around week 26.
- Baby is practicing sucking and swallowing amniotic fluid in preparation for feeding.

Key Appointments and Tests

- 18 to 22 weeks: anatomy scan and checkup
- Potential further genetic testing
- 24 to 28 weeks: glucose screening to test for gestational diabetes

Potential Physical and Emotional Symptoms

- 16 to 20 weeks: Feel baby's movements for the first time
- Increase in energy from the first trimester
- Dizziness
- Heartburn
- Growing breasts and maybe even leaking colostrum (the initial type of breast milk and baby's first food)
- Leg cramps or charley horses in your sleep

Food and Nutrition

- Eat iron-rich foods and consider taking an iron supplement.
- Aim for 75 to 100 grams of protein a day and 1,000 milligrams of calcium to help your baby grow.
- Aim for 25 to 30 grams of fiber and 80 ounces of water (10 glasses) a day to help avoid constipation.

Lifestyle and Self-Care

- Low-impact exercise is recommended: Prenatal yoga, walking, and swimming are great options.
- Get a properly fitting bra as your breasts grow or try a bra extender.
- Plan a babymoon.
- Consider a mindfulness practice, like guided meditation, to relieve stress.

To-Do List

- Start a baby registry and choose a date for your baby shower.
- Let your boss know you're pregnant and make plans for parental leave.
- Order your breast pump (covered by insurance).
- Choose a childbirth class

Signs to Seek Medical Advice

- Vaginal bleeding or leakage of fluid
- Persistent headaches or blurred vision
- Experiencing regular contractions
- If any other concerns arise

General Overview

Your prenatal appointments will increase in frequency in this final stretch. Your care provider will continue to check your vitals and keep an eye out for things like preeclampsia. He or she will make sure baby is growing well, listen to baby's heart rate, and ask how often baby is moving and if you've noticed any changes in movement. Discuss your birth goals and preferences with your care provider and birth partner. Tackle your postpartum to-do list, but don't forget to get plenty of rest too!

Baby Development

- Baby gets significantly bigger, growing from about 2.5 pounds at the end of the second trimester to 6 to 9 pounds by 40 weeks.
- As baby practices breathing, you may start to notice a rhythmic movement—these are hiccups.
- Baby is opening its eyes, sucking its thumb, and getting into position for birth.

Key Appointments and Tests

- 35 to 37 weeks: Group B strep test
- Tour the hospital or birth center where you're planning to give birth
- 40 to 42 weeks: Potential biophysical profile and nonstress test

Potential Physical and Emotional Symptoms

- Linea nigra—a dark line down the middle of your belly
- Stretch marks on your belly, hips, or breasts
- Significant increase in vaginal discharge
- Heartburn
- Shortness of breath
- Mild swelling in feet or hands
- Braxton-Hicks contractions

Food and Nutrition

- Continue healthy eating habits.
- Continue to drink 80 to 100 ounces of water per day (8 to 10 glasses).

Lifestyle and Self-Care

- Incorporate mini stretch routines throughout your day. Squats and lunges are great childbirth preparation.
- Treat yourself to a prenatal massage or a pedicure—or both!
- Use essential oils to promote relaxation and sleep.
- Continue low-impact exercise and mindfulness practice.

To-Do List

- Take a childbirth preparation and an infant CPR class.
- Attend a breastfeeding class or group like La Leche League.
- Get educated on postpartum mood disorders.
- Pack a bag for the hospital or birth center.
- Prepare your home and gather supplies for a home birth.
- Install your baby's car seat.
- Gather baby essentials.
- Gather postpartum recovery supplies.
- Set up postpartum support systems.

Signs to Seek Medical Advice

- Vaginal bleeding or water breaks
- Decline in baby's movements
- Persistent headaches or blurred vision
- Severe swelling
- Going into labor!
- If any other concerns arise

General Overview

You did it; your baby is here! The first twelve weeks of your baby's life are referred to as the fourth trimester. Baby is transitioning from the womb to the outside world and is completely reliant on you for their every need. This is also a huge transformation for you that will come with many ups and downs, and if you aren't well, it's difficult to care for your baby. Keep in mind that the recovery timeline is different for everyone. For many people, healing and adjusting to life with a baby takes much longer than twelve weeks. No matter what your timeline is, it's a gradual process, but you will eventually find a rhythm. Focus on taking care of yourself and your baby, not on "bouncing back" or hitting certain milestones. Reach out for emotional and physical help when you need it, and try to rest whenever you can!

Baby Development

- Your baby will likely lose weight in the first two weeks; loss of up to about 10 percent of their birth weight is expected.
- Four to six weeks: Growth spurt—baby may want to eat more frequently.
- Five, eight, and 12 weeks: Your baby goes through developmental leaps, which can cause sleep regression and extra fussiness.
- Baby may develop cradle cap or baby acne.

Key Appointments and Tests

- First 24 hours: Newborn screening, vitamin K, and eye ointment are offered.
- Three to five days after birth: First pediatrician visit
- Weeks 2, 4, 8, and 12: Pediatrician visits
- Week 6: Postpartum checkup for the birthgiver

Potential Physical and Emotional Symptoms

- If breastfeeding, it can be painful when baby first latches on.
- Breast engorgement and cracked or sore nipples (common in the first couple of weeks)
- Heavy postpartum bleeding, called lochia
- Sore vagina and perineum
- Hemorrhoids
- After a cesarean birth you may experience a sore abdomen; your incision can be painful or itchy too.
- Four to five days postpartum: huge hormonal shift; "baby blues"
- 15 to 25 percent of birthgivers develop a more serious postpartum mood disorder (see page 139).
- Week 6: Your uterus is back to pre-pregnancy size, but your tummy likely isn't.

Food and Nutrition

- Drink lots of water and eat a well-balanced diet, including plenty of fruits and vegetables.
- If you are breastfeeding, it's recommended to get an extra 200 to 500 calories a day.
- If you're breastfeeding, your pediatrician will recommend your baby get a vitamin D supplement. Alternatively, you can take a vitamin that contains at least 6400 IU of vitamin D; evidence shows it will pass on to the baby through your milk.
- See Chapter 12 for information on your baby's nutrition.

Lifestyle and Self-Care

- Self-care and rest for you and your partner should be your top priority after baby's needs are met. Accept help when offered!
- Take a postpartum herb bath or sitz bath to relax and heal your perineum.
- If you're experiencing back or neck pain, make a chiropractic appointment or get a postpartum massage.
- Buy a few new clothes that fit rather than trying to squeeze into pre-pregnancy clothes.

To-Do List

- Sleep when baby sleeps. (No, really. Do it!)
- Reach out to friends and family, a therapist, or a support group for connection and help when needed.
- Plan tummy time for baby.
- If breastfeeding, introduce your baby to a bottle before they are five weeks old so they don't refuse one later on.
- If you are returning to work, make a plan for what work/life balance will look like for your family.

Signs to Seek Medical Advice

FOR YOUR BABY:

- Any fever, even as low as 100.4°
- Excessive sleepiness or not waking up to eat
- Dehydration/constipation (your baby should have five to six wet diapers and three to four poopy diapers a day)
- Yellowing of the skin or eyes
- Infection in umbilical cord
- Infection of the penis from circumcision
- Rapid breathing or wheezing
- Any other concerns that arise

FOR YOU:

- Any fever, even as low as 100.4°
- Discharge or pain/redness around a cesarean scar
- Bleeding that increases or returns to bright red
- Passing clots larger than a golf ball or soaking a pad in less than an hour
- Pain or burning when you urinate
- Vaginal discharge that smells bad
- Signs of mastitis, including flu-like symptoms, fever, and red streaks or lumps in your breasts
- Severe abdominal or chest pain, changes in vision, severe headache, dizziness, chills, or fast heart rate
- Unexplained pain in extremities
- Signs of postpartum mood disorder, including extreme sadness that persists beyond two weeks postpartum
- Any other concerns that arise. Trust your gut feeling and seek help if you're concerned about anything.

"No amount of research, advice, words of wisdom, other parent's experiences, or even prior childcare experiences will tell you how it is going to be to care for this baby. Every baby is different, every parent is different, every day is different. Do the best you can and enjoy your own unique story (no comparisons necessary)."

—Jessica Maki

2

Doctors, Appointments, and Tests

Dr. Emiliano Chavira, MD, MPH, FACOG and Lindsey Meehleis, LM, CPM

In this chapter, we'll discuss different types of care providers and birth locations and how to choose what will be right for you. Our midwife, Lindsey Meehleis, and our OBGYN, Dr. Emiliano Chavira, joined forces to cover everything from what questions to ask at your first appointment to the diagnostic testing that is typical of most pregnancies. Keep in mind that you do have a say in what tests and screenings are performed and you should be an active participant in discussions of your care. Each pregnancy is unique, and you may not need all of the tests outlined in this chapter. Feel free to skip around to the questions that apply to your situation.

Q. How do I know who will be the right care provider for me?

There's no right answer to this question, but a good thing to do is to think about what's most important to you in your pregnancy care experience. Perhaps shared experience is important, so you feel most comfortable with a provider who shares your gender or race. You may prefer someone older, assuming this means more experience. On the other hand, you may feel a younger provider might offer a more modern approach to care. Think about what type of practice appeals to you. Perhaps you would like a smaller practice where you're likely to see one or a small number of providers. A larger practice may mean more choice in providers but could also mean seeing different providers over the course of the pregnancy. Some providers and practices have a technologically oriented approach and like to use tests and medications and other interventions liberally, while others have a more naturalistic or hands-off approach. None of these features are good or bad; trust your instincts. Feeling comfortable with and having trust in your provider are the most important factors in the end.

Q. What's the difference between a doctor and a midwife?

OBGYNs get a general medical-school education and then complete a residency for their specialty in obstetrics and gynecology. The training they receive is focused specifically on complications of pregnancy, so OBGYNs can attend more complicated pregnancies and can perform operative vaginal deliveries (vaginal deliveries with the assistance of forceps or vacuum) and cesarean sections (C-sections). In addition to obstetrics, they also provide gynecology care outside of pregnancy. There are some family practice doctors who get additional training in obstetrics so they can provide prenatal care, and a few of them can even perform cesareans.

Midwives are specialists in the care of uncomplicated pregnancies, and there are a few different ways in which people get their midwife training (see the following question). Midwives have a different approach to pregnancy care compared to doctors. Their training focuses on all the variations and issues related to a low-risk pregnancy. While they do screen for problems and complications in pregnancy, they tend to spend more time on psychological and emotional aspects of pregnancy, healthy lifestyle, family dynamics, and childbirth preparation. They are often interested in empowering pregnant women in their own care and typically use fewer medical interventions compared to doctors. Some midwives independently attend home births or birth-center births, while others work in hospital labor and delivery units alongside OB doctors. A midwife may take care of you for the whole pregnancy, birth, and postpartum period without ever involving a doctor, but they may get a doctor involved if issues arise that require one. Many studies have shown that low-risk birthgivers who receive midwifery care tend to have fewer interventions, lower cesarean rates, and better pregnancy outcomes overall.

Q. What are the different types of midwives, and how do I go about finding one?

There are several different types of midwives, and each state and country has different laws that regulate them.

CERTIFIED NURSE MIDWIVES (CNM)

CNMs go through nursing school and become registered nurses before starting their nurse midwifery training. Many nurse midwifery schools require 18 months to two years of training, and most of this training is done in a hospital setting. Many CNMs are then comfortable with and work in hospital settings. Some, however, seek out-of-hospital experience and offer services at home and in birth centers. Most nurse midwives are regulated by state nursing boards and have tighter requirements of their scope of practice, limiting some choices for their patients. The best place to find a CNM is at the American College of Nurse Midwives (midwife.org).

LICENSED MIDWIVES OR CERTIFIED PROFESSIONAL MIDWIVES (LM OR CPM)

LMs and CPMs have gone through training at schools accredited by either the North American Registry of Midwives (NARM; narm.org) or Midwifery Education Accreditation Council (MEAC; meacschools.org). As laws changed and this education became more formalized, these programs were developed in order to codify the skills needed for this license. These programs usually require three years of in-person training. This type of training does not require in-hospital training and is more focused on the integrative practice of midwifery. While almost all CPMs have training in suturing, giving medications for postpartum hemorrhage, administering antibiotics and IVs, and neonatal resuscitation and have the skills to handle a vaginal breech birth, multiples, and vaginal birth after cesarean (VBAC), not all states will allow midwives to handle these tasks.

LAY MIDWIVES

These midwives obtain all of their skills through the apprentice model with no formal education. Historically, this is how all midwives were trained until education became formalized. In many states, practicing this type of midwifery is against the law, unfortunately, and in most cases, these midwives are not recognized by insurance for reimbursement purposes, so it's important to do your research ahead of time when determining the type of midwife you want.

Q. Are there any questions I should ask when interviewing care providers or during my first appointment?

The short answer is that you should ask all the questions that occur to you to ask, but a few common areas to ask about include:

The structure and policies of the practice. In some practices you will always see the same person, whereas in other practices you may see multiple providers. Ask if the person who sees you for your prenatal care will be the person attending your birth. If you have children, ask if they are allowed at the prenatal visits or if you will need to leave them at home—that alone could determine whether this is the practice for you.

Birth plans. If you have a birth plan, you'll want to review it early on with the provider. Some providers are very respectful of birth plans, whereas others may be outright dismissive. You may not have a specific plan yet, but you might have some general thoughts like "I want a completely unmedicated birth" or "I know I want an epidural." You should share those thoughts early on to see if the provider is supportive of your vision of childbirth.

Doulas. Some parents will hire a doula to assist them during the pregnancy. There are OB providers who do not like to work with doulas, and you will want to find this out early on.

Medical interventions and cesarean sections. A common concern these days is the possibility of medical interventions, including cesareans. Providers vary widely in terms of how they view medical interventions in labor and delivery, so if this is something you have an opinion on, you will want to make sure your views align. You should ask the provider what their C-section rate is, as this can vary wildly from one provider to another. Even midwives will know their C-section rates, even though they don't perform them themselves. If you're carrying twins or have had a previous cesarean, most providers these days will have a strong preference for a repeat cesarean. If these scenarios apply to you and you would like a vaginal birth, then you must discuss this early in the pregnancy. You don't want to find out at the end of the pregnancy that your provider will not support your plan for a vaginal birth.

The main thing is not to be afraid or embarrassed to ask about anything that is really important to you. If you have a lot of questions, prepare a handful of your most important questions for your visit and arrange to address the rest via a phone call, email, or follow-up visit. But you should always expect to have all of your questions answered and pay attention to the provider's attitude when responding. They should be an active listener and not be dismissive or make you feel like your questions aren't valid.

Q. What are the chances that the doctor I choose will be the one available when I go into labor?

This really depends on the specific practice and how it is structured. You might envision seeing the same person at each prenatal visit who will also attend your birth. This scenario is becoming less and less common among OB practices. Most modern practices involve coordination of care among a group of providers, which may be composed of a mix of OBs, midwives, physician assistants, or nurse practitioners. Some neighborhood prenatal clinics only provide prenatal care and don't do deliveries. They usually have an arrangement with one or more local hospitals where their patients will go for the birth itself. Although group practices are becoming increasingly common, you may still be able to find a small private practice in your area where you see a single provider or a small group of providers.

If you choose midwifery care for a planned home or birth-center birth, you're much more likely to be cared for by the same person or a small team throughout your pregnancy, including the birth.

Q. How do I know if I'm a good candidate for a home birth or birth-center birth?

Out-of-hospital birth is a reasonable option for most people who experience an uncomplicated pregnancy. In simple terms, this means the pregnant person has no significant medical conditions that might impact labor, there are no major birth defects in the baby, and the pregnancy progresses to full term. Most home births and birth-center births are attended by midwives, although there are a small number of doctors who attend home births as well.

Criteria for out-of-hospital births vary by state, but the midwives themselves are meticulous about making sure you're an appropriate candidate for either home birth or a birth-center birth. For pregnancies with potential complications—including carrying multiples, breech presentation (where the baby is positioned bottom-down), or a history of previous C-sections—the availability of out-of-hospital birth will vary depending on state law.

Also, out-of-hospital births are unmedicated, so if you're pretty sure that you're going to want an epidural in labor, then out-of-hospital birth is probably not for you. That said, many people change their views as they learn more about pregnancy and childbirth, so it's always worthwhile looking into these options with an open mind.

Q. What can I expect at my OBGYN appointments?

The first few visits will likely be the most involved. In addition to detailed paperwork, a complete physical exam is usually performed to see if there are any health concerns that will need to be addressed. At one of your first visits, a Pap test is done if you're due for it as well as a blood panel and urine tests to check your blood type and to screen for anemia and various infections such as HIV, hepatitis B, and other sexually transmitted infections.

Subsequent visits tend to be short follow-up visits. Every appointment will start with taking your vital signs and a urine test, mainly to check for protein. After about 20 to 24 weeks of gestation, there will usually be some sort of assessment of fetal growth. In most cases this will mean placing a tape measure over your belly and measuring from your pubic bone to the top of your uterus to make sure the uterus is growing as expected. In some practices the size of your baby may be measured with an ultrasound. You will usually be asked if the baby is moving normally, which is typically felt around 20 weeks. In addition, you will usually be asked about the three universal warning signs in pregnancy: uterine contractions, leakage of fluid, and vaginal bleeding. If you have any of those symptoms, your provider will ask you about it in greater detail to determine whether it is truly a concern. Beyond that, this will be your chance to ask questions about things that have come up since the last visit. There may also be discussion about other issues such as planning details about the birth, breastfeeding, and postpartum contraception.

At various points during prenatal care, some standard tests are either recommended or offered, including fetal ultrasounds (see pages 22-23) and genetic tests (see page 27), all of which are typically completed by 20 to 22 weeks gestation. Between 24 and 28 weeks, a blood test for gestational diabetes is conducted (see page 29). Around 36 to 38 weeks, a vaginal/rectal swab will be taken to test for group B streptococcus (GBS; see page 32).

Q. What can I expect at my midwife appointments?

Most midwife appointments, much like appointments with an OB, include a general well-being check, which includes checking your blood pressure; a urine test; questions about swelling, headaches, visual disturbances, and fetal movement; and assessing the baby's position using Leopold's maneuvers, which are done by palpating your belly. Most midwives also offer assessment through ultrasound and blood work. For many midwives, an emotional check is just as important as the physical check, so they'll talk with you and your partner to assess stress levels, emotional well-being, nutrition and fluid intake, quality of sleep, recommended supplements, exercise, and more. Some midwives, myself included, also make it a point to discuss fears about the birth, the changing dynamic of the family, and other physical and emotional changes. If you don't have a care provider giving you this care, I recommend bringing some of these things up yourself and building a relationship of trust and respect.

Q. How often can I expect to see my doctor or midwife?

In typical prenatal care, the appointments in the first trimester are spaced further apart, occurring every three to five weeks. Around 28 weeks, the frequency of appointments increases to every two weeks. After 36 weeks, visits are scheduled weekly. This is a general framework; visits may occur more often than this in certain complicated situations like gestational diabetes or hypertension, for example.

Q. Are there any red flags I should look out for that would indicate my provider's biases about birth?

Some pregnancy care professionals try to minimize interventions, while others have a lower threshold for introducing interventions like induction of labor, episiotomy, and C-section. If your personal views about pregnancy are very different from your provider's views, this is a red flag for difficult conflicts over the course of your pregnancy. A provider who brings up interventions like induction of labor or cesarean repeatedly or early in the pregnancy when there is no real reason to mention them may be more inclined to utilize these procedures at the end of the pregnancy. Certainly, if a provider has a very high cesarean rate, this may be an important clue. The Healthy People 2020 project has recommended a first-time cesarean rate under 24 percent. The World Health Organization, on the other hand, suggests that the ideal cesarean rate is between 10 and 15 percent. You can use these numbers as a general frame of reference, but know that a provider with a high C-section rate may not necessarily be "scalpel happy." For example, an OB who works in a practice with midwives may be referred all the patients with complications in pregnancy or childbirth, so they may be handling a set of patients who are already at high risk for C-section.

Another issue is paternalism, or an attitude of "the doctor knows best." Modern approaches to care are more interactive, and patients these days should have much more say in how their care plays out. Unfortunately, you're likely to run into many paternalistic providers. If you find that a provider seems rude or arrogant, interrupts you a lot, or doesn't seem to take any of your concerns seriously, these may be red flags. This is not to say that a provider should always agree with you and accept everything that you want, but your concerns should always be listened to and addressed respectfully. Although it may be uncomfortable to do so, you should express how you're feeling and give your provider an opportunity to change. If these types of interactions keep happening, then you might be better off trying to find another practice that suits you better.

Q. What is a perinatologist (maternal-fetal medicine specialist), and why would I need one?

A perinatologist is a doctor who has completed a general OBGYN residency program and an additional fellowship training program in maternal-fetal medicine (MFM). MFM training focuses on the care of complicated pregnancies, whether from a maternal health condition such as diabetes, heart disease, kidney disease, cancer, etc., or because the baby has a birth defect or other problem that needs to be addressed. A previously uncomplicated pregnancy may become complicated if unexpected problems arise, such as preterm labor or preeclampsia.

The predominant reason you might be referred to a perinatologist is when your pregnancy is complicated by maternal or fetal conditions. In some cases, only a consultation is required, and the perinatologist will make recommendations to your original provider for your care. Depending on the issue, the MFM specialist may see you more than once over the course of the pregnancy. In some cases, the pregnancy is complex enough that the original provider will transfer your care completely to the MFM specialist.

Because perinatologists are experts at pregnancy ultrasound, a person with an uncomplicated pregnancy may be referred to an MFM just for an ultrasound. Sometimes people are referred to MFM offices for genetic counseling and discussion of genetic testing options.

Q. When will I get to see my baby on an ultrasound?

Some practices perform an ultrasound at the start of prenatal care to count how many babies you're carrying, to confirm your expected due date, and to look at some basic fetal anatomy. However, this isn't automatically done in all practices and could be optional if a physical exam indicates that the size of your uterus matches how many weeks along you think you are based on your last menstrual period.

It has become standard these days to offer a nuchal translucency (NT) ultrasound when the fetus measures between 11 weeks and 14 weeks and two days. At the NT ultrasound, which is really a genetic screening test, you can see some major details like the brain, heart, spine, arms, and legs. If the images are very clear, you may even be able to see some fingers and toes.

After that first-trimester ultrasound, it's fairly standard to have another ultrasound at 18 to 22 weeks. This is sometimes referred to as the anatomy ultrasound or anatomy scan. At this time, your baby is substantially larger, and you can usually see much more detail in the face, heart, spine, kidneys, hands, feet, and other organs. This ultrasound is a detailed examination of your baby and is used to spot any major birth defects. Also, measurements are taken of the head, belly, and upper thigh to see if your baby is growing normally. If you want, you might be able find out the baby's sex, assuming that clear images of the genitalia are obtained.

Q. Should I get a 3D or 4D ultrasound?

There is currently very little medical purpose for 3D and 4D ultrasound. There are some practices that incorporate 3D or 4D imaging into medical care, particularly if associated with academic centers, but these would be the exception. For routine medical purposes, 2D ultrasound is currently the standard. 3D and 4D ultrasounds are done mostly for entertainment purposes, so it is up to you whether you want to have one of these ultrasounds performed. There is a guiding principle in obstetric ultrasound known as the ALARA principle, which stands for "as low as reasonably achievable." Essentially, while ultrasound is considered safe in pregnancy, ultrasound exams should be limited to no more than necessary and should be used thoughtfully, cautiously, and responsibly.

Q. When will I find out my baby's sex?

It's possible to find out your baby's sex from genetic tests and ultrasound exams. Genetic tests are usually done for pregnancies that are at increased risk for chromosomal conditions like Down syndrome or other genetic conditions and not for the sole purpose of determining fetal sex. One form of genetic testing is a noninvasive prenatal test or screen (NIPT or NIPS), which is a blood test. This can be performed as early as 10 weeks. Beyond NIPT, there are two diagnostic tests: chorionic villus sampling (CVS) in the first trimester and amniocentesis in the second (see page 28 for more on amniocentesis). Again, because these are primarily genetic screening tests, you should carefully weigh the pros and cons of doing them.

Ultrasound is the other way of determining the fetal sex. Keep in mind that in the first trimester, genitalia can appear indistinct, so the risk of error is higher. It is usually at the fetal anatomy ultrasound, performed between 18 and 22 weeks, where an attempt is made at determining the fetal sex. The accuracy of second trimester ultrasound for fetal sex determination depends on how clearly the genitalia are visualized as well as the skill and training of the person who is performing the ultrasound.

As a side note, if you don't want to know the sex of your baby or don't want your baby assigned a gender at birth, make sure your care provider knows your preference. It's also not a bad idea at the start of every visit and ultrasound exam to remind your care provider or ultrasound tech of this. Also note that in the United States, all newborns must be assigned a binary gender marker on birth certificates.

Q. What are some reasons my pregnancy might be considered "high risk"?

There is no universally agreed-upon threshold for when the term "high risk" should be used. As a result, many people may hear that their pregnancy is "high risk" and then overestimate how high the risk actually is. Because the word "high" is subjective, it cannot communicate the actual magnitude of the risk in a numerical way.

This can make the pregnancy much scarier and more stressful than it needs to be.

However, there are certain factors that might qualify a pregnancy as high risk. One is preexisting maternal medical conditions that have the *potential* to affect pregnancy, including diabetes, hypertension, lupus, heart disease, or kidney disease. Specific birth-related medical conditions that can develop during the pregnancy, like gestational diabetes, venous thromboembolism (blood clots forming in the veins), or preeclampsia can affect you, too. If you have a history of risk in a prior pregnancy, such as preterm birth, preeclampsia, a previous cesarean, or complications during childbirth, you may be classified as a high-risk pregnancy again. Finally, a pregnancy might be deemed high risk for reasons related to the baby rather than the mother, like major malformations or physiological problems like severe anemia.

Q. What do I need to be aware of with regard to prenatal care as a plus-size person?

Prenatal care and childbirth ideally should be no different for a plus-size person than for anyone else. Statistically, there may be a slightly higher chance of certain issues in pregnancy like gestational diabetes, preeclampsia, and even cesarean birth. Statistically, a plus-sized person also has a higher chance of birthing a bigger baby, but this is by no means a forgone conclusion. If your care provider is telling you that you're "high risk" or that you'll need a cesarean solely based on your weight, look for another provider. The sites PlusSizeBirth.com and SizeFriendly.com are both great resources for questions to ask when interviewing providers.

Ideally, you can make some changes to your diet and start a regular exercise plan *before* getting pregnant. But keep in mind it's not really about the numbers on the scale—it's the healthy habits and feeling strong that are most important. If you're already pregnant, focus on healthy food choices and regular exercise. Many worry about the safety of exercise in pregnancy, but research shows that people who exercise in pregnancy actually have better outcomes than people who do not. See page 82 for more on exercising in pregnancy. There are published guidelines regarding how much weight you should gain during your pregnancy, but obsessing about weight too much can be overly stressful. Some weight gain will be beyond your control, as people vary in how much water they retain, how much their breasts grow, etc. That's why it is preferable for pregnant people of all sizes to focus more on healthy habits than on weight itself. If the number on the scale is stressing you out at your checkups, face away from the scale and let your provider know that you do not wish to discuss your weight.

Q. What prenatal tests/screenings are available to me? Do I have to get them all?

The standard prenatal tests include:

Blood Typing. Your blood type is checked in case you have the need for a blood transfusion. Your Rh status is also tested to determine whether you're Rh-positive or Rh-negative. Most birthgivers who are Rh-negative should receive a Rhogam injection at around 28 weeks to prevent them from developing antibodies against Rh-positive blood in case the baby is Rh-positive. After birth, another dose of Rhogam may be given if the baby is found to have Rh-positive blood. An antibody screen is also performed to see if you have already formed red blood cell antibodies, either from a prior pregnancy or from a prior blood transfusion.

Rubella immunity. You will also be tested for rubella immunity; if you're found to be rubella nonimmune, vaccination after the pregnancy is over is recommended.

Complete Blood Count (CBC). The three main elements of the CBC are the white blood cell count, the red blood cell count, and the platelet count. If you're found to be anemic (low red blood cell count), your care provider will determine what type of anemia is present and whether it needs to be treated. The most common type is iron deficiency.

Tests for several sexually transmitted infections. These include HIV, herpes, syphilis, hepatitis B, gonorrhea, and chlamydia. It's critical to discover whether any of these infections is present so measures can be taken to reduce the chances of passing the infection to your baby during childbirth.

A Pap test. This should be done early in pregnancy if you're not already up-to-date. Some people may worry that the Pap test may pose risk to the baby, but you can rest assured that the test is safe at any time during the pregnancy.

Urine cultures. These are routinely done in early prenatal care because bacterial overgrowth in the urine is common in pregnancy and, if discovered, is important to treat to avoid serious kidney infections and other complications.

You have the right to decline any test that you wish; however, there are no really good reasons to skip them.

Q. Genetic testing: What are the advantages and disadvantages of having it done?

There are a variety of genetic tests that may be offered to you along the way. Since each test has its own pros and cons, they should be considered individually. Whether you choose to have these tests done is a personal decision, and you can opt in to some while declining others.

Genetic tests during pregnancy can be divided into two types: testing for conditions in the pregnant person that could be passed on to the baby and testing the baby directly for genetic conditions. Testing the pregnant person involves blood tests to see whether gene conditions such as cystic fibrosis or spinal muscular atrophy are present. The exact conditions tested for depend on the pregnant person's family history and ethnic background. Genetic screening for the baby mainly tests for Down syndrome and a short list of other genetic conditions. Screening tests are easy because they're simple blood tests, but they have a known rate of false results, so they cannot be considered 100 percent accurate. Diagnostic tests are procedures that obtain a sample of either the placenta or the amniotic fluid. These results are highly accurate but come with a very small risk of causing a pregnancy loss. Most people with an average-risk pregnancy choose to start with a blood test. Diagnostic tests are usually done if the baby has a higher risk of having a genetic condition—for example, if a screening test is positive or if fetal abnormalities are seen on an ultrasound.

The main advantage of genetic testing is to have more information so that you can make decisions based on that information. If you're found to be a carrier of a particular condition, further testing can be done to see if the baby has inherited that condition. If a serious condition is diagnosed in the baby, you can choose to terminate the pregnancy or begin preparing to care for a child with a serious genetic condition. The main disadvantage of genetic testing is the anxiety that may be caused by positive test results; note that you can decline any and all genetic testing.

Q. What's an amniocentesis, and why would I need one?

An amniocentesis (amnio, for short) is a diagnostic test in which a sample of amniotic fluid is collected via a needle inserted into the uterine cavity under ultrasound guidance. The amniotic fluid is then sent to a lab to have any number of tests performed. These advanced tests give much more detailed and accurate genetic information about your baby compared to a blood test like the NIPT.

If your NIPT test indicates the presence of a chromosomal condition in your baby (like Down syndrome, for example), an amniocentesis is typically the next step to confirm the diagnosis. In cases where a fetal malformation is seen on ultrasound, an amniocentesis for advanced genetic testing will likely be offered to you. While it is always your choice whether to have an amnio, in cases where a malformation is present, getting one is advisable.

Another reason to consider an amnio is to see if the baby is affected by a known genetic condition in your family. Whether to have an amniocentesis in a situation like this is a very personal decision. One question to consider in this scenario is what, if anything, you would do with the information during the pregnancy. This could include either medical therapy for the baby or termination of the pregnancy. If there is nothing that you would do, then it may not be worthwhile pursuing this testing during pregnancy. But if you think that you will experience a lot of anxiety and stress worrying about this issue, then you might decide to have the testing done just for peace of mind. While there is a very small risk of an amnio causing a pregnancy loss, studies indicate that this risk is about one pregnancy loss per every 400 procedures. This risk, even though it is small, explains why amniocentesis is typically only performed in pregnancies that are at increased risk for fetal genetic conditions.

Q. What is the glucose test, and when will I have it done?

The glucose test checks for the presence of gestational diabetes mellitus (GDM), a pregnancy-specific form of diabetes that is caused by hormonal changes. This test is done between 24 and 28 weeks. If you already have diabetes, then you should not have this test. It is only for those who have not been diagnosed with diabetes prior to the pregnancy. GDM will disappear after the pregnancy ends, although it may be a warning sign that you're at increased risk for developing regular diabetes in the five to 10 years after the pregnancy. Diabetes is a very important issue in pregnancy because the high blood sugar in your body exposes your baby to abnormally high levels of glucose, which can cause a wide range of serious conditions, miscarriage or stillbirth, and excessive growth of the baby, potentially leading to serious injuries at birth as well as increasing the chances of a C-section.

In the United States, the most common method of conducting the glucose test is to drink a 50-gram glucola drink. Your blood sugar level is checked at fasting and then one hour later. If your blood sugar is normal, then no further testing is done. If your blood sugar is elevated, you may or may not have GDM, and a three-hour test is ordered to make the diagnosis. For this test, a 100-gram glucola drink is given. Your blood sugar is checked at fasting and at one-, two-, and three-hour intervals. If two or more out of the four values are elevated, you have GDM and your provider will begin treatment, usually involving medication along with diet and exercise changes. If only one value is elevated, then technically you do not have gestational diabetes, but your provider may want you to follow a strict diet and exercise plan and may even ask you to check your blood sugar. Sometimes an early glucose screen is done in the first trimester if you're at higher risk of developing GDM. If the early glucose screen is normal, then it should be repeated at 24 to 28 weeks to see if gestational diabetes has appeared later in the pregnancy.

Q. Count the kicks: What are fetal kick counts, and how do I do them?

Fetal kick counting is a formalized process for counting how many times your baby moves within a specified time frame, usually after 28 weeks. A common method is to pick the same time of day (usually when you know baby is active) and count fetal movements (anything from a roll to a kick to a punch) and report how long it takes to get to 10. Other methods may be recommended by your pregnancy care provider. In theory, this functions as a test of fetal well-being that you can do at home. There is some debate about how to incorporate fetal kick counts into prenatal care and their ability to prevent pregnancy complications, and as such there are differences in what providers recommend, with some providers never bringing fetal kick counts up. If it feels like a reassuring thing for you to do at home, feel free. You can find more information (and a free app) at CountTheKicks.org.

Q. Why might I need a nonstress test or biophysical profile?

The nonstress test (NST) and biophysical profile (BPP) are both tests of fetal well-being, much like fetal kick counts. The ultimate goal of these fetal monitoring tests is to prevent cases of stillbirth if possible. An NST involves attaching an ultrasound device to the mother's belly to detect the fetal heart rate and monitor it for 20 minutes, although it can be longer if there are any questions about the first 20 minutes. The BPP is an ultrasound examination that looks at the amniotic fluid volume as well as fetal tone, movement, and breathing. A full BPP may require observing the baby with ultrasound for up to 30 minutes. There is also the modified BPP, which entails checking the amniotic fluid volume with ultrasound and performing an NST. These tests of fetal well-being are collectively referred to as antepartum fetal surveillance or antepartum testing. If any of these tests are found to be abnormal, your care provider may request additional monitoring or possibly referral to the hospital. If the test results are sufficiently concerning, delivery of the baby might be recommended.

Antepartum (third trimester) tests are not routine for all pregnancies; they are usually performed in complicated pregnancies where the risk of stillbirth is thought to be higher than average. The other time they are common is when a pregnancy goes past the estimated due date. The downside to antepartum testing is that NSTs and BPPs are known to have a fairly high rate of false positive results, or false alarms. This could lead to a baby being inappropriately delivered too early based on abnormal antepartum testing results, and there can be serious consequences from early delivery, so these decisions must always be made thoughtfully. While there are no high-quality studies that definitively prove that antepartum testing does more good than harm, this is a very firmly established component of prenatal care for women with complicated pregnancies.

Q. Should I tour the hospital or birth center? What questions should I ask?

Taking a tour of the hospital where you will give birth is a great idea. It will allow you to figure out exactly whe re you're supposed to go so that in the whirlwind of labor you know where to park, how to enter the hospital, etc. In addition, most hospital tours will give you an orientation to the birth process specific to their center and will cover useful details, including where labor and delivery is, where postpartum recovery happens, visiting hours policies, whether the rooms are private or shared, what you can and can't bring, rules regarding photography and filming in childbirth, what tests are done for the newborn, the process for getting the birth certificate, and checkout procedures. If you think you may want an epidural, this is a good time to find out whether the hospital has an anesthesiologist on the labor and delivery unit available to provide immediate service to laboring people or if they have one on call but not necessarily stationed in the hospital. In general, you will have the opportunity to ask nonmedical questions related to the facility, the labor and delivery unit, the staff, and any policies and procedures around the birth process.

Q. What is the group B streptococcus (GBS) screening?

Group B streptococcus is one of the many bacteria that may be living in a healthy person's body under normal circumstances. It usually does not cause harm to the person carrying it. During pregnancy, we pay special attention to GBS because, in about 2 percent of cases, it can be transmitted to the baby, making the baby very sick. The current recommendation is to screen almost all women for GBS between 36 and 38 weeks. The screen is performed by swabbing the lower vagina and rectum with a cotton-tipped swab. If you had a baby infected with GBS in a prior pregnancy or if GBS is found in your urine culture in early pregnancy, then you're considered a GBS carrier and the screening is not done. In pregnant people who are considered to be GBS carriers, antibiotics are given during labor to reduce the risk of infection in the baby.

Q. What's a cervical exam, and why would I get one during pregnancy?

When people refer to a cervical exam, they are usually talking about a digital exam in which the care provider inserts their fingers into the vagina to feel the cervix. With a digital exam, you can feel things like the position of the cervix and whether it is soft or firm. You can assess whether the cervix is long and closed or whether it's starting to efface (thin out) or dilate (open). The cervix can also be examined by inserting a speculum into the vagina to look at the cervix or through either a vaginal ultrasound, where an ultrasound wand is inserted into the vagina, or with an ultrasound placed on the lower belly.

In the middle of pregnancy, you may have a cervical exam if there are any symptoms of preterm labor. After 37 weeks, some providers will offer a routine cervical exam to see whether you're beginning to dilate. Some providers feel that this is not necessary and do not do these routine cervical exams. When you show up to the hospital and think you might be in labor, a cervical exam will be offered to see if your cervix is dilating. While you're in labor, additional cervical exams may be offered to monitor the progress of your cervical dilation. Of note, midwives often do fewer cervical exams in labor than OB doctors do, as they tend to use other ways of judging your progress. It is always your right to refuse a cervical exam and is something you should discuss when choosing your care provider. For some, a history of sexual abuse contributes to their desire to avoid cervical exams.

"Everyone talks about symptoms like nausea and vomiting, exhaustion, tender breasts, and how this means your pregnancy is totally normal! I wish someone would also say that you can also have a totally healthy pregnancy without any of the 'typical' pregnancy symptoms. It's worrisome when you think you should be having a symptom and you're not. But it doesn't mean anything is wrong. It could just be your normal!"

—Sarah Moyer

3

Physical and Emotional Symptoms

*Lindsey Meehleis, LM, CPM
and Courtney Butts, LMSW*

Most pregnancies come with at least a few symptoms, and others have a long list of them. This chapter will cover what to expect when it comes to the most common ones. There's so much variation between pregnancies, so feel free to jump ahead to the questions that are relevant to you. Our midwife, Lindsey Meehleis, will cover the physical symptoms first, and then we will turn it over to our mental health expert, Courtney Butts, to cover potential emotional symptoms. Keep in mind these are all "variations of normal," and if you have any concerns, you should always consult with your care provider.

Q. If it's called morning sickness, why is it lasting all day?

A little bit of trivia: Old wives' tales used to refer to the trimesters of pregnancy as the morning (first), afternoon (second), and evening (third). So, in this case morning refers to the first trimester, which is the most common time nausea is experienced during pregnancy—and it often occurs throughout the day and night. According to the American Pregnancy Association, up to 85 percent of people experience some form of digestive discomfort, including nausea, indigestion, and bloating, in the first trimester. About 65 percent of people experience vomiting in their first trimester.

Q. Is it normal to have this much vaginal discharge?

The amount of vaginal discharge in pregnancy can be quite alarming, but rest assured, copious amounts of vaginal discharge are normal. It's typically white and milky and shouldn't smell bad. Use a panty liner—not a tampon—and let your care provider know if it is a color other than white or clear, smells bad, or is causing pain or itchiness.

Q. I'm throwing up all the time! Is my baby getting enough nutrients?

When you're constantly throwing up, it's hard to imagine you have any nutrients left. But be assured your body is prioritizing your baby, so they are getting the nutrients they need to grow (even if it's at your expense). First trimester sickness may seem like it will never pass, but typically the second trimester will bring relief and you'll have a chance to make up for this time and replenish yourself when you're feeling better. However, in extreme cases, your care provider may offer medications or other protocols. (More on hyperemesis gravidarum on page 168.)

Q. When does nausea typically ease up?

This is different for everyone. Some people notice symptoms for only the first few weeks, and some experience symptoms throughout the pregnancy. The average pregnant person will only experience symptoms throughout the first trimester. Remember that these symptoms and how you're feeling are a variation of normal, so try to not compare yourself to your sister or your neighbor or even your last pregnancy—each pregnancy is different.

Q. I'm exhausted! Why do I feel like I have zero energy?

You're growing major organs, tiny eyelashes, and little baby toes—it takes work! Your body is working around the clock to provide for your growing baby, and it can take a toll. Give yourself grace and a lot of reassurance that what you're feeling is normal. I know you're likely busy, and it can be hard to find time for rest, but do what you can to take it slower and make time for yourself without guilt; you're growing an actual human being!

Q. I keep getting headaches. What can I do?

Headaches are usually hormone-related but can also be complicated by dehydration and low blood sugar. If you're having recurring headaches, make sure you're getting enough water (aim for 10 eight-ounce glasses of water a day). If you aren't eating because everything sounds horrible, try just a couple bites of something every couple of hours to help keep your blood sugar up. If you're still getting headaches, they are likely hormonal, just like the headaches you might get right before your period. One way to treat symptoms naturally is by using essential oils topically on the places of discomfort. The easiest, most accessible one is peppermint oil. You may also take Tylenol (see the Medications Chart on page 204).

Q. I'm experiencing some cramping in my lower abdomen. Is that normal?

"Normal" is a funny word in pregnancy. While there are several different variations of normal, care should be individualized. Get to know your body and see what's normal for you. If you're ever truly worried, consult with your care provider. However, here are some general guidelines.

IN THE FIRST TRIMESTER

In the first trimester, cramping is usually caused by your growing uterus. By the end of your first trimester, your uterus has reached the size of a grapefruit and lifted out of your pelvis. If your cramping is associated with vaginal bleeding or intense pain, please contact your care provider. This could indicate a potential miscarriage or ectopic pregnancy. While this information is not intended to cause fear, knowledge is power. Knowing what your body is doing will empower you because most of the time, abdominal cramping is just uterine growth.

IN THE SECOND TRIMESTER

In your second trimester, the cramping in your uterus is typically caused by your round ligaments stretching to accommodate your growing uterus. If you notice cramping that is rhythmic and getting stronger and closer together, call your care provider. The top two causes for preterm labor are dehydration and stress. So, if you're noticing preterm labor symptoms and more than 10 Braxton-Hicks contractions in one hour, drink a big glass of water first and see if this soothes your uterus.

IN THE THIRD TRIMESTER

In the third trimester, cramps are usually increasing Braxton-Hicks contractions to get your uterus ready for birth. The same precautions from the second trimester apply here. You may also notice cramping after the baby engages or drops in your pelvis preparing for birth. This can irritate your uterus and can cause contractions for a few hours. In my midwifery practice, I ask my patients to take a calcium magnesium supplement (following the dosing on the bottle), an Epsom salt bath, and a double dose of fish oil (again, as listed on the bottle) to relax their body and uterus, but be sure to check with your care provider.

Q. Help, I can't poop! How do I deal with constipation in pregnancy?

This is a common complaint of pregnancy. One of the most important things you can do is eat a well-balanced diet with lots of fiber and stay well hydrated, but if that alone isn't working, check with your care provider about supplements to help with constipation. I recommend my clients take a calcium magnesium supplement to keep things moving, as magnesium is a muscle relaxant and will help you maintain healthy bowel movements during pregnancy. Start with the recommended dosage on the bottle and increase the dosage by a half-dose each day until you get loose bowels. Once you have reached loose bowels, go back to your dose from the day before. The dosage you need might change throughout your pregnancy as hormones fluctuate and affect your GI tract differently, so just listen to your body.

Q. Is diarrhea in pregnancy normal?

Yes. Again, we have hormones to thank for this massive change to your gastrointestinal (GI) tract. A person's pH balance changes throughout the course of the pregnancy, and a change in the alkalinity or acidity of the intestines leads to either diarrhea or constipation, and it can be hard to find the balance in between. Too much diarrhea can lead to dehydration, so if you have diarrhea for more than four to five days, be sure to contact your health care provider.

Q. I noticed blood when I wiped. Should I be concerned?

Blood at any point in pregnancy except in labor tends to alert and concern expectant parents—this is completely understandable!

IF YOU'RE IN YOUR FIRST TRIMESTER

In the first trimester, blood can mean a couple of things. Bright red vaginal bleeding can be an indicator of miscarriage but not always. Common causes of bleeding and spotting in the first trimester are implantation bleeding (when the fertilized egg attaches to your uterus) or a subchorionic hematoma, which is a small accumulation of blood in the uterus that typically resolves itself with no other complications but still has to come out. Sometimes, spotting is the result of low progesterone levels. Regardless, with first trimester bleeding, you should always contact your care provider.

IF YOU'RE IN YOUR SECOND TRIMESTER

The most common causes of bleeding in the second trimester are sex or constipation that causes popped capillaries when you strain. It usually goes away after a couple of hours and is nothing of concern. However, if you're experiencing heavy bleeding or it's accompanied by Braxton-Hicks contractions, get in touch with your care provider. Another cause of bleeding in the second trimester can be a low-lying placenta or placenta previa, so if you've been diagnosed with this and are experiencing vaginal bleeding, let your care provider know.

IF YOU'RE IN YOUR THIRD TRIMESTER

Bleeding in the third trimester is also usually due to sex or constipation. However, as you near your due date, the culprit is usually cervical change from dilation or "bloody show," which is mucus tinged with blood from ruptured blood vessels in your cervix—a good sign that your cervix is effacing and dilating. It's possible to experience "bloody show" for weeks or not at all. If you're concerned, contact your care provider.

Q. I'm experiencing some swelling. Should I be concerned?

Some swelling is normal because the blood volume in your body increases by about 50 percent when you're pregnant. So it's not uncommon to notice some swelling, like the rings on your finger getting tight or your feet swelling up a bit. However, excess swelling is not normal. If you're experiencing extreme or sudden swelling, especially in your hands and face, get in touch with your care provider to check your blood pressure and rule out preeclampsia.

A "normal" amount of swelling is sometimes due to a lack of protein in your diet (I recommend 75 to 100 grams a day) or dehydration (get plenty of water!). Other factors that can contribute to swelling are heat, a lack of movement, or too much activity, such as a really long walk or standing for a long period of time. It is also a common thought that swelling is caused from too much salt, but in fact, in pregnancy adding extra high-quality sea salt or Himalayan pink salt (not table salt or salty processed foods) to your diet can help with mineral absorption and actually reduce swelling.

Q. Why am I having such bad heartburn? Are there any remedies?

Heartburn can occur at any point in a pregnancy, but it is most common from the second trimester on, when pregnancy hormones relax the valve of your esophagus, allowing stomach acid to escape. Toward the end of your pregnancy, as your uterus grows to accommodate your baby, all of your organs shift up and out of the way, which puts pressure on your stomach, slowing the digestion process. There are a few ways to ease heartburn, including eating several small meals a day; avoiding spicy, acidic, and fatty foods; and eliminating alcohol and caffeine. Other natural remedies include eating a teaspoon of Manuka honey after meals and taking digestive enzymes like papaya enzyme pills. If your heartburn is severe, your doctor can prescribe medication.

Q. My back is killing me! Is this common?

Common, yes . . . normal, no! Yes, your body is changing and expanding, but there is no reason to walk around in pain when there are options for treatment. Around the seventh month of pregnancy, you start to release a hormone called relaxin, which softens and relaxes the ligaments in your pelvis. This is great as your pelvis opens to accommodate the birth of your baby, but it can cause back pain. If you're in pain, seek out a Webster-certified chiropractor. You can find one in your area by searching the International Chiropractic Pediatric Association website (ICPA4Kids.com).

Q. What is sciatic nerve pain, and how can I treat it?

Sciatic nerve pain is pressure on the sciatic nerve in your pelvis, which causes shooting pain down your legs—sometimes quite significant pain. This is usually caused by an imbalance of the pelvis, and the best way to treat this pain is with a Webster-certified chiropractor (see the previous question).

Q. What's this dark line going down the middle of my stomach?

This line is called the linea nigra, which is caused by hormonal changes that can alter the pigment of your skin. You may also notice darkening of the skin on your face, nipples, armpits, and vagina. Not everyone gets this line or skin darkening, but if you do, it's totally normal, and there's nothing you can do to change it.

Q. I keep having shooting sensations in my pelvic floor. What's going on?

This is commonly referred to as "lightning crotch" and usually occurs when baby starts to engage into your pelvis, pushing on nerves that cause "shooting pains" down into your pelvic floor. It can be startling and super uncomfortable, though it's quite common. Once your baby is born, it will improve as the pressure in your pelvis is relieved.

Chiropractic adjustments and pelvic-floor physical therapy can help but don't always take away the sensations depending on the baby's position.

Q. Why is my face breaking out? I normally have clear skin.

Just like teenage acne, pregnancy acne is due to hormonal changes. It can often be worst in the first trimester, and as the hormones balance in the second trimester, your face should also start to clear up. Routinely cleaning your face before bed will help. You can also use organic essential oils to help—tea tree oil to treat your pimples, lavender oil to help them heal, and frankincense oil to reduce scarring.

Q. Is it normal to have insomnia during pregnancy? How can I get better sleep?

Insomnia is normal! Still, it's important to consider *why* you're not sleeping. If you're wide awake because of anxiety, then finding ways to reduce and cope with stress is important. If you're wide awake with back and hip pain, then figuring out how to ease that pain is a good idea (see page 42). Your body may also be helping you prepare for a baby who will need to be fed at all hours of the night. Something you can do to get better sleep is to make sure that you have a good bedtime routine. Limiting use of electronic screens, drinking a warm cup of tea, and taking magnesium all might help you sleep better.

Q. What is considered normal weight gain?

The recommended weight gain for a "typical" pregnancy for an "average" sized person is listed on the American College of Obstetricians and Gynecologists' website (ACOG, acog.org). With that said, since each person starts pregnancy at a different weight—and some people experience drastic morning sickness and lose weight, while others must have carbs to get them through and gain weight—it isn't practical to place strict guidelines on weight gain. Stay healthy, eat whole foods, avoid processed sugars and carbs as much as possible, and feel healthy and strong within your body, regardless of what the scale says.

Q. I'm hot all of the time. Is that normal?

Your basal metabolic rate actually goes up by 20 percent in pregnancy due to the increased blood supply, which is why you generally run hotter. This is totally normal.

Q. What changes can I expect with my breasts during pregnancy?

Get to know your breasts! They can change so much throughout your pregnancy and then again after delivery. Your glandular tissue grows to accommodate the upcoming lactation, so they may feel sore and tender. Your nipples may also change colors and grow as well. The change in pigment is actually so your baby has a dark area to "aim for" because babies can't find the nipple without assistance.

Q. What is perinatal depression and anxiety, and how do I know if I have them?

Depression or anxiety occurring during pregnancy or within one year after delivery is known as perinatal depression or anxiety. These illnesses, also known as perinatal mood and anxiety disorders (PMADs), impact up to a third of new parents. It is well known that new parents can feel anxious or overwhelmed by the transition into parenthood, and meeting your baby can evoke many different emotions. However, when these thoughts interfere with daily functioning, it's important to seek help. Onset of symptoms can be sudden or gradual, and they can include:

» Agitation
» Anger/rage
» Sleeping either too little or too much
» Feeing restless or irritable

» Changes in appetite
» Feeling sad or depressed, crying a lot, or all three
» Little interest in being a parent
» Feelings of worthlessness or guilt
» Thoughts of wanting to be dead, suicide, or wanting to just disappear
» Headaches, dizziness, numbness, or hyperventilation
» Feeling empty, numbness, or nothing at all
» Intense fear
» Trouble focusing, remembering things, or making decisions

Perinatal depression and anxiety can bring about intense feelings that interfere with a person's ability to care for themselves and their baby. Risk factors include a history of anxiety or depression, lack of access to resources, and exposure to trauma or complications in pregnancy, birth, or breastfeeding. For people of color, these risk factors are compounded by isolation, lack of social support, stigma, and chronic environmental stressors. If you feel you may be experiencing PMADs, you are not to blame. PMADs are treatable with professional help. If you're experiencing any of these symptoms, please speak with your care provider about treatment options.

Q. If I have a history with depression or anxiety, am I more at risk for developing a perinatal mood disorder?

One of the biggest factors to predict depression and anxiety in a pregnant person is previous history. If you have had depression or anxiety in the past, you may be vulnerable to experiencing them during pregnancy or the postpartum period. Previous history also includes familial history of perinatal mood and anxiety disorders or symptoms during pregnancy. Also, personal or family history of depression, anxiety, bipolar disorder, eating disorders, or obsessive-compulsive disorder (OCD) may put you at further risk for developing a perinatal mood or anxiety disorder.

Q. Is it possible to prevent perinatal mood disorders?

While it may not be possible to prevent perinatal mood disorders, you can set things in place to lower your risk. One of the best ways to prevent mood disorders is to identify and build your support network. Fulfilling relationships with those around us help us feel more connected and supported. These relationships may include family, friends, neighbors, or a doula. Many communities have support groups for birth parents, partners, and extended family; connecting with others in a similar life phase can feel supportive. Another way to reduce your risk is to seek professional help. A licensed mental health professional can help you sort through your feelings and develop healthy coping techniques. Childbirth education can help you prepare for birth and your new life after baby arrives. Creating a birth plan as well as a postpartum plan can be helpful in managing expectations. Additionally, educate yourself about the signs and symptoms of perinatal mood and anxiety disorders and where to seek help if needed.

Q. Is it safe to take antidepressants during pregnancy?

Yes, there are safe options available. Exposure to medications during pregnancy may carry some risk, but for some medications the risk is minimal. Untreated mental illness can pose serious risks to the pregnant person and the baby. All treatment decisions are made on a case-by-case basis and should include a risk/benefit analysis with your medical provider.

Q. How do I find a therapist who specializes in perinatal mental health?

Postpartum Support International has a list of providers who specialize in perinatal mental health (postpartum.net). Your care provider may also have recommendations for perinatal mental health providers in your area.

Q. My anxiety is through the roof. What are some things I can do to ease it?

Pregnancy and parenthood can bring about concerns and worries you never thought about before. Most new parents are anxious or worried about some aspect of pregnancy, birth, or parenthood. One way to ease anxiety is to develop relaxation skills, including progressive muscle relaxation, diaphragmatic breathing, and guided imagery. Mindfulness, yoga, and meditation can also help. You can also look at your diet—eating more nutrient-dense foods may help lessen anxiety symptoms. Exercise reduces the levels of the body's stress hormones, so step outside and take a brisk walk. If your fears or worries leave you unable to concentrate in your daily life, it may be time to reach out to a mental health professional and work with them to uncover the underlying causes of your anxiety and develop healthy coping and problem-solving skills.

Q. How do I mentally prepare for childbirth?

Mentally preparing for childbirth is a smart thing to do. Some ways to do so include the following:

» Do research and ask questions. This will help you feel more empowered throughout your pregnancy.
» Hire a doula.
» Focus on positive experiences when reading stories and watching videos.
» Practice relaxation techniques.
» Develop affirmations or mantras.
» Talk to your partner and support team about your needs and desires.

All people have the need to feel connected. If you aren't feeling supported by your partner, family, or friends, it's okay to communicate your wants and needs. A few good ways to do so are:

Use "I" statements. An "I" statement allows you to talk about how you feel instead of attacking or blaming the other person. For example, "I feel frustrated when I attend prenatal appointments by myself."

Focus on the root of the issue. It can be tempting to talk about everything that is going wrong; pinpoint what you want or need from your support team and focus on those desires.

Communicate exactly what you want and need. Saying "I want you to be more supportive" leaves too much room for interpretation. Instead, you could say, "I would like for you to attend the next prenatal appointment with me."

Seek out additional support. Consider hiring a doula or attending a pregnancy support group in your area.

Q. *I'm a survivor of sexual trauma and worried about how this will come up during my pregnancy and birth. What should I do to prepare?*

Trauma is a subjective, emotional response to an event that rewires the brain and how we see the world around us. Research shows that emotions associated with prior trauma (such as physical, emotional, or sexual abuse) can resurface during labor and delivery. Working through your past trauma with a mental health professional is a good first step. Sharing your trauma history with your health care provider can be helpful so that you can talk through possible triggers. Also, hiring a trauma-informed doula or birth assistant can help create space for you to feel more informed and empowered during your pregnancy, birth, and the postpartum period.

"The difference between the stomach bug and morning sickness in my mind? When you're pregnant, you throw up and immediately go eat another meal because you're SO. DANG. HUNGRY!"

—Jillian Dilbeck

4

Common Illnesses and Ailments

Dr. Emiliano Chavira, MD, MPH, FACOG

In addition to the symptoms you're experiencing due to fluctuating hormones, you may also have questions regarding how to address common illnesses when you're pregnant. Dr. Chavira will go over the most frequently asked questions when it comes to getting sick while pregnant. Please use this as a guideline and, as always, consult with your medical provider for diagnoses and treatment.

Q. How is a common cold treated during pregnancy?

Rest and drink plenty of fluids. Wash your hands frequently and minimize contact with others as much as you can to limit the spread of infection. If you have a prenatal appointment, it would be best to call and reschedule so as to avoid exposing other pregnant people in the waiting room to your cold.

There are over-the-counter remedies that you can take to ease the symptoms of the common cold, which is caused by a virus and does not require antibiotics. For fever or pain, Tylenol (acetaminophen) is safe. There is a chart of medications that are safe for pregnancy on page 204, and your care provider will have this information as well. For a stuffy nose, you can use a first-generation antihistamine, or if you prefer to avoid medications altogether, you can also use a sinus rinse.

Q. What happens if I get the flu while pregnant?

The flu in pregnancy is usually similar to the flu outside pregnancy. For most healthy adults, the flu will get better on its own within a few days, although there is an antiviral medication that can make the illness shorter and less severe. See your care provider to confirm whether the symptoms you're experiencing are the flu or the common cold. If you do get the flu, your care provider can prescribe an antiviral medication specifically for influenza, like Tamiflu (oseltamivir). Ideally you should start this medication within two days of onset of symptoms. You may also treat flu symptoms as you would the common cold (see the previous question). Among pregnant women who get the flu, a small percentage will get severely ill, possibly even requiring a hospital stay, and an even smaller number of pregnant women die from the flu every year. In severe cases, preterm birth can occur. Because of these risks, most doctors recommend you get the flu vaccine at the start of the flu season as a preventive measure. If you can't keep any fluids down, are dizzy, have difficulty breathing or chest pain, or are experiencing regular uterine contractions, go to the ER for evaluation.

Q. I have terrible allergies! Can I take any OTC medications?

Over-the-counter antihistamines are safe in pregnancy (see the Medications Chart on page 204). First-generation antihistamines like Benadryl (diphenhydramine) are preferable to second-generation antihistamines like Claritin (loratadine) and Zyrtec (cetirizine), though the latter can still be used. You can also try a nasal spray like Flonase (fluticasone) or Rhinocort (budesonide). Note that these nasal sprays do not provide immediate allergy relief; it usually takes a few days or so for them to fully kick in. Sometimes, these nasal sprays can dry out your nasal passages and lead to nosebleeds. In this case, you can use a simple nasal saline spray to keep your nasal airways moist.

Q. Is there anything I can take for a sinus infection while pregnant?

If you're feeling sinus congestion with a lot of nose stuffiness, you can try to relieve the congestion with nasal rinses, antihistamines, or nasal sprays (see the Medications Chart on page 204). If you have an ongoing runny nose and congestion with facial pain for 10 days or more or if you have a fever, you should see a medical professional. If sinusitis is diagnosed, treatment will involve getting rid of the congestion so your sinuses can drain and eliminating the infection. Decongestants like pseudoephedrine and phenylephrine are best avoided in pregnancy unless absolutely necessary. Common antibiotics, like amoxicillin, clarithromycin, or azithromycin, can be prescribed to help eliminate the infection. All of these are considered safe for use in pregnancy.

Q. *What happens when you get food poisoning while pregnant?*

Food poisoning in pregnancy is generally similar to food poisoning outside pregnancy. Most mild cases of food poisoning are caused by common viruses. Symptoms usually include nausea and vomiting followed by watery diarrhea. There may or may not be a low-grade fever. Make sure to drink plenty of fluids until the infection passes. If you cannot keep fluids down or if you feel light-headed or dizzy, you should go to the hospital for IV fluids. Most mild cases of food poisoning will have no harmful effect on the baby, as your placenta protects the baby against most infections. But some infections, like listeriosis and toxoplasmosis, have the ability to harm the baby.

Bacterial gut infections cause nausea, vomiting, and diarrhea just like viral gut infections, but the additional warning signs that the infection might be bacterial include high fever, abdominal pain, and blood or mucus in the stools. Bacterial gut infections tend to be more serious than viral infections and are treated with antibiotics. If you have any of the warning signs for bacterial food poisoning, you should call your care provider or go straight to the hospital.

Q. *How will I know if I have a yeast infection, and what treatment should I get?*

Vaginal yeast infections are very common, and while they can be quite bothersome, they are generally not dangerous to you or your baby. Typical symptoms include vulvar itching, burning, or both with a curdy white discharge. There is usually not much of an odor. You may also feel burning when you urinate. If you have been diagnosed with a vaginal yeast infection in the past and the symptoms are the same or if what you're experiencing matches this description, it's a safe bet you're dealing with a yeast infection. Treatments are over-the-counter antifungal creams like Monistat (miconazole), Canesten (clotrimazole), or Gyno-Trosyd (tioconazole). They come in various formulations from one day to seven days of treatment, and any of these is fine. If you try one of these treatments and the symptoms do not go away, then you should see your care provider for an exam. Sometimes a yeast infection can be confused for other conditions, like chemical irritations or other types of infections.

Q. *What are the signs of a UTI or a bladder infection during pregnancy? Is it bad for the baby?*

Most people use the term UTI (urinary tract infection) for what is actually a bladder infection. The typical signs of a bladder infection (cystitis) in pregnancy include pain or burning during urination or right after. You may have to urinate much more frequently than normal, and you may feel intense urgency, that is, the sensation of needing to urinate comes on suddenly and severely. Sometimes when you have a bladder infection you will have the urge to urinate but then very little actually comes out. Although urine with an unusual or strong odor is not generally a reliable symptom of a bladder infection, bad or strong-smelling urine may warrant a test to look for infection.

For a typical bladder infection, the bacteria are very unlikely to enter into the uterine cavity, so the baby should not be directly affected by a UTI. However, if a bladder infection progresses to a more serious condition like a kidney or bloodstream infection, this could potentially lead to a preterm birth. If you experience symptoms of a bladder infection, call your care provider.

Q. *Will I know if I have a kidney infection? How?*

A kidney infection is a serious illness. If you have a kidney infection, you will feel quite ill, with a fever and back pain, which can be severe. The pain will be slightly off to the sides of your midback (slightly higher than the level of your belly button). You may also have nausea and vomiting, and you may feel uterine contractions. Most kidney infections will respond quickly to IV antibiotics, but you can expect to spend at least a couple of days in the hospital. In severe cases, the infection can spread to the bloodstream. Also, severe kidney infections can lead to preterm birth. If you're diagnosed with a kidney infection, you will be admitted to the hospital and started on IV antibiotics right away. When you're discharged, you will probably be sent home with a prescription for several more days of antibiotics to treat the infection completely.

Q. My ear is really bothering me. Are ear infections common in pregnancy?

Ear infections may be slightly more common in pregnancy due to swelling of your airway lining, which can block the eustachian tube (the tube that drains the inner ear). This causes the feeling that your ears are plugged up, muffled hearing, and sometimes ear pain or even an ear infection. Try a saline sinus rinse, an antihistamine, or a nasal corticosteroid spray to reduce this swelling and unblock the ear (see page 53). If the pain continues or worsens or if you have a fever or drainage from the ear, see a care provider who can look in your ears to see if you have an ear infection. Some ear infections are viral and should improve on their own. If a bacterial infection is suspected, then antibiotics will be prescribed.

Q. What medications can I take (or not take) while pregnant?

Always check with your care provider before taking any medications during pregnancy. The few that are known to cause birth defects or other harm to the fetus should be strictly avoided. Another type of medication to be wary of is medications that are new to market and likely do not have enough research evaluating their safety in pregnancy. Because of this, medications that have been around longer and have more safety research behind them are usually favored for use in pregnancy. Some medications fall into a sort of gray zone. In these cases, the decision whether to take them will depend on how necessary or beneficial they are in your specific situation. Reference the Medications Chart on page 204 for a list of common medications and whether they are safe in pregnancy and postpartum. MotherToBaby.org is a good resource for quality information about specific medications and other exposures in pregnancy.

Q. For what reasons would I be put on bed rest?

Bed rest is an old-fashioned therapy that has been prescribed for things like bleeding in the first trimester, symptoms of preterm labor, a shortened or dilated cervix, placenta previa (when the placenta is down low in the uterine cavity covering the uterine cervix), and multiple gestations in the hopes of reducing the chance of miscarriage, preterm labor, or stillbirth. You should be aware, however, that bed rest has become an outdated practice. Studies have failed to show that bed rest helps to prevent or even delay preterm birth. In fact, some studies have shown an *increased* risk of preterm birth when bed rest is prescribed. There are other potential harms from bed rest including weakened physical condition, body pains, the formation of blood clots in the legs or lungs, and psychological distress or depression.

The ACOG has now formally recommended against bed rest for the prevention of preterm birth in its most recent guidelines. If your pregnancy care professional recommends bed rest to you, it would be a good idea to ask some questions. You'll want to get explanations about exactly what type of activity restriction is being suggested, for what reason exactly, for how long, and whether any studies exist that show that this intervention will be helpful.

"One of my favorite parts about being pregnant is the food cravings. Both pregnancies, I had an intense craving for pepperoncinis, and I ate at least half a jar a day. I bought out the entire supply at our corner store."

—Erin Danial

CHAPTER

5

Food and Nutrition

Lindsey Meehleis, LM, CPM

Since everything you put into your body during pregnancy will also be nourishing your growing baby, it's natural to have questions about what is and isn't safe to consume. Beyond that, you're likely wondering how to optimize your nutrition to keep you feeling good and help your baby grow and develop. In this chapter, our midwife, Lindsey Meehleis, will address the dos and don'ts of nutrition as well as some goals to make sure you're getting all of the vitamins and nutrients you and your baby need.

Q. I'm vegetarian/vegan. Can I continue my regular diet while pregnant?

Yes. The nutrients some vegetarians and vegans struggle with getting enough of during pregnancy are protein and iron. It's recommended you get between 75 and 100 grams of protein every day, so if you're worried that you might not be getting enough, be sure to log your food and add quality proteins as needed. Additionally, you will want to be sure you're getting enough iron in your diet, at least 27 milligrams a day. Eat lots of leafy greens and consider an iron supplement if needed. Floradix is a great plant-based iron supplement that can help increase your iron levels without causing constipation. Interestingly, many vegetarians and vegans will start to crave animal protein throughout their pregnancies. So, if you're craving it, I encourage you to listen to your body. You can certainly return to your pre-pregnancy diet as soon as you no longer have those cravings.

Q. Can I continue my keto, paleo, or gluten-free diet?

Yes. In fact, excessive and "empty" carbs turn into sugars in the body, which can cause a number of issues including the potential for a bigger baby. That said, often plain white carbs (e.g., toast, pasta, crackers, rice) are about all you can keep down during the first trimester. Don't worry too much about your diet; just listen to your body and try to maintain a balanced diet high in protein, fruits, and vegetables.

Q. How much protein do I need daily?

As your baby gets bigger, your body needs more nutrients to help it grow, and protein is good for baby's brain development. Aim for 75 to 100 grams of protein each day. Hard-boiled eggs or a protein drink are an easy way to get a protein boost early in the day. It's also a good idea to keep protein-rich snacks with you on the go, as eating small amounts throughout the day can help with digestive issues—good options are nuts, string cheese, carrots and hummus, or protein bars.

Q. *My care provider mentioned my iron levels are low. What can I do to increase them?*

Low iron is not an uncommon side effect of pregnancy. It's estimated that your blood volume almost doubles to nourish your baby and accommodate for the blood loss following birth. When there is an expansion in blood volume, there has to be a dilution, causing your hemoglobin or iron level to decrease. Be empowered throughout your care, and ask your care provider for copies of your labs. If you start to feel run down with extreme fatigue or shortness of breath, you may have a low hemoglobin number, often 11.5 or less. If you're starting your pregnancy with a lower level, try to increase your iron intake right off the bat. Eat iron-rich foods, including dark leafy greens, meat, eggs, beans, and bone broth. You can also take an iron supplement like Floradix.

Q. *Is spicy food bad for me or the baby?*

There is no evidence that suggests spicy foods are bad for your baby. If you crave spicy food, eat it. However, it can contribute to heartburn, so pay attention to whether it affects you.

Q. *What are the best foods to eat during pregnancy?*

The best way to eat throughout your pregnancy is intuitively. The first trimester may be a time where you're very limited to foods that your queasy stomach can tolerate. Try to avoid processed foods as much as possible and eat foods that are whole, fresh, non-GMO, and organic when possible. Stick to the outer perimeter of the grocery store. What you're looking for are healthy fats (nuts and seeds, avocados, and certain fish, like salmon), 75 to 100 grams of protein a day, fresh veggies and fruits, and lots of hydration.

Q. *Are there any foods to avoid while I'm pregnant?*

Limit your intake of fish that are high in mercury, such as king mackerel, shark, swordfish, and tuna. It is also advisable to avoid raw or undercooked meats and seafood, raw or unpasteurized dairy, soft cheeses, lunch/deli meats, raw or undercooked eggs, and unwashed vegetables and fruits. The best way to eat during pregnancy is intuitively. If something doesn't taste good or doesn't make you feel good, don't eat it. This is your body and your baby; do your research and make a conscious educated decision as to what is right for you.

Q. *I live for my morning coffee. Is any amount of caffeine okay during pregnancy?*

The general consensus is that one small cup of coffee a day is fine. There is conflicting data, and the March of Dimes states that until more conclusive studies are done, pregnant people should limit caffeine intake to less than 200 milligrams per day. This is equal to about one 12-ounce cup of coffee. If you decide you want to eliminate coffee during your pregnancy but miss the ritual, you can try switching to decaf coffee or tea.

Q. *I know I need to take a prenatal vitamin, but how do I know which one to take?*

This is tricky because it's hard to make a blanket statement about what each person needs. Folate, or vitamin B9, is important for a growing baby's cell development, so in addition to eating leafy greens and foods rich in folate, you'll want to find a prenatal vitamin with methylated folate. Folic acid is the synthesized form of folate, often found in fortified foods. Some people have genetic mutations that cause their bodies to have difficulty breaking down folic acid, so studies point toward methylated folate as the better choice.

Q. *Are there any additional vitamins I should be taking?*

In addition to a healthy diet and a good prenatal vitamin, I recommend taking 5,000 IU (international units) of vitamin D and a probiotic daily and getting a source of essential fatty acids, like fish oil or, for vegetarians, hemp, chia, or flax seeds. These can be taken straight or mixed into a smoothie of your choice. Other supplements and vitamins may be recommended based on your history, so talk to your care provider about which ones will be safe for you.

Q. *What about herbal supplements? Can they cause miscarriage? Which ones should I avoid? Are there any herbal supplements that will support me during pregnancy?*

The FDA does not regulate herbs and other supplements, and thus, there is no official research on their uses in pregnancy. Err on the side of caution, and consult your care provider before taking any. If herbal supplements are something you want to use in your pregnancy and your doctor isn't familiar with the subject, you can also consult an herbalist, a naturopath, or another care provider who is more knowledgeable.

In terms of herbs to avoid, stay away from black cohosh and blue cohosh as they can cause uterine contractions (some midwives do use them to induce labor). Parsley, taken in medicinal doses, has been linked to miscarriage (don't worry—the amount you find in food is fine).

As for herbal supplements that can be helpful, I recommend liver supplements to my pregnant clients because your liver supports your pregnancy and growing uterus. Good herbs to support your liver are dandelion root, nettles, and yellow dock. You can buy these in tincture form or buy bulk herbs and make herbal infusions. Adding red raspberry leaf will help with taste, and it is an excellent herb for your uterus. An easy recipe is to put two ounces of nettle leaf, two ounces of red raspberry leaf, and two ounces of yellow dock in a mason jar, fill with hot water, and steep overnight. In the morning, drain and drink throughout the day. Again, this is what I recommend in my own practice, but I suggest that you consult with your care provider before trying this.

Q. I know that I should avoid alcohol, but I've also heard that the occasional glass of wine is fine. What's the deal?

There aren't many good studies on the effects of alcohol consumption in pregnancy and whether there is a "safe" amount. We *do* know that alcohol enters the fetal bloodstream and that significant amounts of alcohol are detrimental to the baby. The CDC, ACOG, and the American Academy of Pediatrics all advise that no amount of alcohol is safe during pregnancy, so the prudent thing to do is to abstain entirely. However, in other countries you may find different norms. As a practitioner who addresses both physical and emotional aspects of pregnancy, I encourage my clients to address the root of why you might like a glass of wine. If it's for stress reduction, explore other ways to minimize stress, like taking a warm bath or going for a long walk, which will continue to be helpful as you move into parenting. We recommend the book *Expecting Better: Why the Conventional Pregnancy Wisdom Is Wrong—and What You Really Need to Know* by Emily Oster for more on this subject.

Q. Should I be eating organic or non-GMO foods?

The long-term effects of GMO and pesticide-treated food are still unknown. I do encourage you to eat organic and non-GMO foods as much as possible, especially with organic foods becoming more readily available, including at budget-friendly stores like my favorite—Trader Joe's. Visit your local farmers' markets or farms to find good deals, and budget as best as you can.

Q. *I drank alcohol or smoked, or did both, before I knew I was pregnant. Will my baby be okay?*

This is a very common situation to find yourself in, and it's difficult to make a blanket statement without specifics like how long until you knew you were pregnant, how much you were drinking/smoking, etc. But rest assured, most of the time, your baby will be just fine as long as you begin healthy habits as soon as you know you're pregnant. If you're concerned, follow up with your care provider.

Q. *I was partaking in recreational drug use before I found out I was pregnant. Will it affect my baby?*

Again, it's difficult to make a blanket statement about this because the answer will depend on what type of drug, how heavy the use, and how long you used it for. The most popular recreational drug in the United States is cannabis, and some states have legalized it for medical or recreational use. The ACOG notes that there are concerns around impaired neurodevelopment as well as exposure to the adverse effects of smoking and as such discourages the use of cannabis during pregnancy and nursing. If you were using any recreational drugs before finding out you were pregnant, it is recommended that you cease immediately and check in with your care provider.

"I didn't have many cravings,
but the aversions—hoo boy!
I got very familiar with the
bathroom of my grocery store.
The first time I puked there, it
was because I walked by the
cheese section. The second
time it was the olive bar. The
third time it was the BAKERY
of all things. I had a woman
ask me if I was okay from the
next stall over. I replied, 'Yes,
just pregnant,' in between
heaves. She laughed and said
'Congratulations! And I'm
so sorry!'"

—Sara Martin

Environment, Lifestyle, and Self-Care

Bryn Huntpalmer

Becoming pregnant can feel like an open invitation for advice from everyone in your life, including complete strangers. In this chapter, we will go over some of the most common questions that may come up regarding your environment and your daily habits and lifestyle. To be thorough, I will give you as much information as I can, though in general, I err on the side of caution, especially when the available research isn't clear on the subject. If you want to take a deep dive into the research and evidence around the dos and don'ts of pregnancy, I recommend reading *Expecting Better: Why the Conventional Pregnancy Wisdom Is Wrong—and What You Really Need to Know* by Emily Oster.

Q. *I've heard that I should avoid cats while pregnant. Is that true?*

Nope. The reason you've heard this is because of something called toxoplasmosis, which is a rare parasitic disease that cats sometimes carry, and, if contracted, it can be harmful to your baby. Cats get this disease from eating raw animals, so if you have an indoor cat, it's unlikely that your cat will become infected. Even if your cat gets the parasite, you can only become infected from their feces, so you would have to touch their feces and then touch your mouth without washing your hands. (Gross!) To be vigilant, simply have someone else change the cat's litter or wear gloves while you do it.

Q. *What do I need to know about taking care of a pet while pregnant?*

Aside from being aware of the potential for cats to carry toxoplasmosis, there's not much that needs to change regarding taking care of cats and dogs while pregnant. If you have a large or unruly dog that pulls on a leash, you may want to have someone else walk it so you don't have any unexpected falls. It's also a great idea to help your pets prepare to meet your baby by bringing them around other babies/toddlers during pregnancy. You can also have someone bring a blanket with baby's scent on it for your pets to smell before you arrive home with your baby.

However, if you have a small rodent—like a hamster, guinea pig, or mouse—you could potentially be exposed to a virus called lymphocytic choriomeningitis (LCMV). This virus can cause severe birth defects and even miscarriage, so it's best to avoid cleaning cages and contact with their saliva, urine, blood, and droppings. Reptiles can carry salmonella, so avoid touching them, and if you do, be sure to wash your hands and any surfaces they've been in contact with.

Q. How does indoor and outdoor pollution affect my growing baby?

Outdoor air pollution isn't good for anyone but can be especially concerning for pregnant moms. If you live in an area where pollution is a regular concern, the best thing to do is check the air quality by going to AirNow.gov before spending a lot of time outside. If the air quality is poor, follow the guidelines listed on the site. For example, you may be instructed to stay inside as much as possible or avoid exercising outdoors.

Perhaps surprisingly, indoor air quality is of bigger concern. According to the Environmental Protection Agency, Americans spend 90 percent of their time inside, and air pollutants are often two to five times higher indoors. Now is a good time to focus on reducing indoor air pollution as much as possible. Swap out toxic products for ones made from natural ingredients; use ventilation when cooking, cleaning, or using things that put off fumes like paint or hairspray.

Have your home inspected for mold or asbestos if you live in an area where those toxins are common. Finally, be sure you have a carbon monoxide detector on each level of your house. An air purifier can help remove smoke, mold, germs, and allergens from your air—consider placing one in your bedroom where you likely spend more time than other areas of your house.

Q. I want to paint the baby's nursery. Are there certain paints I should avoid?

Painting while pregnant likely poses very little risk to your baby, but there aren't any actual methods of measuring degrees of toxicity. If this is something that will stress you out, have someone else paint the nursery for you! If you decide to paint, it's always a good idea to ventilate the room and avoid using spray paint or other solvent- or oil-based paints. Most paints on the market for household use are going to be fine, but look for paint with low or zero VOC (volatile oil compounds) to add a layer of precaution. Additionally, avoid refinishing old painted furniture, and be sure to test the existing paint in the nursery as well if you live in an older home. Much paint manufactured before 1978 contains lead, and breathing that in can be very toxic to your and your baby's health.

Q. Are traditional household cleaning products bad for my baby? What natural alternatives can I clean with?

In short, yes. There are several studies that show babies born to women who held jobs where they used cleaning products regularly had babies with higher risks of birth defects or long-term health issues like asthma. Plus, as discussed on page 69, indoor air pollution is a real concern, so if you can remove any products with known toxins from your home, it's going to be beneficial to your whole family's health. Unfortunately, the United States doesn't closely regulate or test the chemicals in our household and personal-care products.

A good way to investigate the products in your home is to use the product search function on the Environmental Working Group's website (EWG.org) or the Think Dirty app. These tools can also help you find better alternatives. It's also really amazing how much vinegar and baking soda can accomplish when cleaning. There are lots of DIY recipes online for making your own cleaning products with natural ingredients. You'll likely end up saving money, and you'll have peace of mind knowing exactly what is in them.

Q. Can I burn candles during pregnancy?

Yes, but it may not be the best idea. Again, there is little regulation around what goes into candles in the United States, and burning petroleum-based paraffin candles releases toxins into the air, contributing to that pesky indoor air pollution. Additionally, many candle wicks emit carcinogens when lit. If you really want to burn candles, look for an all-natural soy-based candle that is free of dyes, chemical binders, artificial fragrances, and phthalates. You should also make sure you're ventilating your home when burning candles and limit the number of hours per day that you're burning them.

Q. Are essential oils safe to use during pregnancy?

Essential oils are distilled from plants and have the fragrance of the plants from which they come. Aside from smelling good, many of them have medicinal uses such as helping with aches and pains, nausea, or stress. Unfortunately, there is very little regulation in the United States about what goes into essential oils that you find on store shelves, so they could have synthetic fillers and other unknown ingredients. You'll want to find a reputable brand and talk to your care provider before starting to use essential oils. Start slowly, with diffusing and topical use, and don't ingest essential oils while pregnant. There are a few oils, including wintergreen, clary sage, hyssop, birch, rosemary, and camphor, that should be avoided during pregnancy, so do your research first. Many midwives and aromatherapists use essential oils in the care of pregnant women and to aid in labor.

Q. Is it okay to use bug spray?

With the recent concern over Zika virus, you might be wondering about bug spray. Zika is a mosquito-borne illness that has serious negative effects on a growing fetus. Protecting yourself from Zika should be your top priority if you live in an area where it is commonly found. The Environmental Working Group recommends a bug repellent with picaridin at a 20 percent concentration or DEET with a 20 to 30 percent concentration.

There are some potential side effects of using chemical repellents, so they should be used as directed and in moderation. If you live in an area with a large mosquito population, especially if Zika is present, it's a good idea to take additional precautions like staying indoors as much as possible when mosquitos are out, wearing long sleeves and pants, and ensuring that mosquitos aren't entering your home by keeping doors closed and windows screened. Zika is not currently locally transmitted in the United States, so you will likely only have to worry about it if traveling abroad. It is recommended to avoid traveling to places with Zika outbreaks if at all possible. You can find areas with Zika via the CDC Zika Travel Information site.

If you have to travel to an area with Zika, take every precaution to avoid being bitten by a mosquito.

Q. How does cigarette or cannabis smoke affect my baby? What if someone I live with smokes?

Smoking tobacco during pregnancy has negative effects on your baby, including preterm birth, low birth weight, and birth defects like cleft lip or cleft palate. Smoking around a newborn also increases the risk of sudden infant death syndrome (SIDS), and nicotine has negative impacts on a baby's developing brain and lungs, so e-cigarettes and other tobacco products are also off the table. Unfortunately, secondhand smoke carries all of the same potential risks as if you were smoking. If someone you live with smokes, have them do so outdoors and remove their outer clothing before coming back in as cigarette residue also has harmful effects for you and your baby.

There isn't a lot of research yet around marijuana use during pregnancy, but until we better understand short- and long-term effects, the ACOG and CDC both advise against marijuana use while pregnant. If you have used or are currently using marijuana for medicinal reasons, consult your care provider. As far as secondhand cannabis smoke, you're probably okay if you're in a well-ventilated area like an outdoor concert or large building. If you live with someone who smokes cannabis, ask them to smoke outside.

Q. I can't get comfortable in bed. What's the best position to sleep in?

As your uterus gets bigger and heavier, it puts pressure on the vena cava (a large vein that carries blood to your lower half). Doctors recommend that pregnant people sleep on their left side to prevent this compression. It's fine to sleep on both sides throughout the night, but try to avoid sleeping on your back as much as possible. A body or pregnancy pillow between your legs can make the side-lying position more comfortable.

Q. Should I take pregnancy photos?

Documenting this time in your life is a wonderful idea. The best time to have pregnancy photos taken is between 30 and 34 weeks. Your bump is big enough to be the star of the photos, but you aren't so big that you're overly uncomfortable. You'll want to book a photographer well before 30 weeks, though, because many will fill up their schedules in advance.

Q. Is it okay to dye my hair? What about perms or chemical hair straightening?

Hair coloring is generally considered safe during pregnancy. It's recommended to wait until after the first trimester so that a baby's vital organs and functions are formed; as an extra precaution, consider using natural dye or getting highlights or balayage instead of all-over color so that the dye isn't coming into direct contact with your scalp. As for perms or chemical hair straightening, again, wait until after the first trimester and make sure you're in a well-ventilated area. For all of these hair treatments, try to stretch out the time between appointments so you aren't going as often.

Q. Is it okay to get a tattoo during pregnancy?

The main concern with getting tattoos during pregnancy is the risk of contracting an infection. If you're visiting a reputable tattoo artist, this risk is very small, but it's still recommended to wait until after pregnancy to get a tattoo—again, erring on the side of extra precaution. A safer, temporary alternative is a henna tattoo that lasts up to a month. Many pregnant people choose to have it applied to their bellies. Make sure you're using a natural, safe henna, and avoid black henna—it contains paraphenylenediamine (PPD), which can cause burns and blistering. Be sure to read all labels.

Q. Are piercings allowed while pregnant?

It's recommended to avoid getting piercings on your belly button, nipples, or genitalia during pregnancy due to the changes your body will go through. Piercings in other areas also carry risks if they become infected. If you're determined to get a piercing while pregnant, make sure you find a reputable, licensed piercing studio and strictly follow guidelines for taking care of your piercing.

Q. What should I know about getting my nails done while pregnant?

Manicures and pedicures are generally considered safe during pregnancy, but it's recommended to limit the amount of chemicals you're exposed to, so try to space out your visits. Make sure you choose a clean salon that uses sterile instruments and doesn't share them between customers. Finally, try to find a well-ventilated nail salon or one that uses nontoxic products.

Q. Is any amount of time in a hot tub or sauna allowed?

Your body temperature should never rise above 102.2°F while pregnant. Many hot tubs are set to 104°F, which can cause your body temperature to rise above 102.2°F in just 10 minutes. If you can lower the temperature of your tub and limit your time to 10 minutes or less, you can enjoy a short soak. Drink water and get out immediately if you start to feel light-headed or show signs of dehydration. Saunas range in temperature from 140°F to over 200°F, so they should definitely be avoided!

Q. If I take a hot bath, will I "cook" my baby?

Nope! But use caution, of course. As long as your body temperature doesn't rise above 102.2°F, baths are safe. That said, baths are a safer option than hot tubs because your upper body is likely above water, and the temperature begins to cool off the longer you sit in the tub.

Q. What should I know about traveling and vacationing while pregnant?

Planning a fun vacation during pregnancy will give you something to look forward to, but there are a few things to keep in mind:

Timing. In general, you'll want to be close to home toward the end of your pregnancy in case you go into labor. It's not recommended to fly after 36 weeks, and many airlines will require a doctor's note if they suspect you're in the final weeks of pregnancy.

Destination. The location you choose for your vacation deserves some consideration as well. For example, if you aren't used to high altitudes, it can be an even harder adjustment when pregnant. Also, many foodborne illnesses are more common in certain countries and can cause complications for your baby.

Skip the cruise. Aside from seasickness and being in the middle of the ocean should you need medical care, cruises are also known for outbreaks of sicknesses like norovirus.

Stay hydrated and keep it moving. Whether you're taking a road trip or flying, it's a good idea to stay hydrated and to take breaks to stretch your legs and move around a bit—even if that's just taking a walk down the aisle of a plane.

Take it easy. Be prepared to take it a little easier than you're used to—jet lag, extra time on your feet, and dehydration are common travel concerns that will be amplified when pregnant.

Remember your medications. Don't forget to pack any medications you're taking as well as your prenatal vitamins.

Q. Are there any activities I should avoid on vacation?

If you're typically an adventurer, it can be hard to sit back and relax by the pool during vacation! While there are plenty of activities you can enjoy, you should avoid high-impact activities or those with a risk of falling (for example, surfing, skiing, and horseback riding). Most tourism companies will let you know when certain activities are off-limits during pregnancy, and it's best to abide by those recommendations.

Q. Can I benefit from chiropractic care during pregnancy?

Pregnancy can bring on many new aches and pains in your body thanks to hormonal changes and the added weight you're carrying around in your abdomen. Chiropractic care can help to ease discomfort and adjust your pelvis, which can help your baby get into an optimal position for birth. You'll definitely want to find a chiropractor who is specifically trained in prenatal and postnatal work. You can go to ICPA4Kids.com and do an advanced search to find a chiropractor who is trained in the Webster Technique.

Q. Can I get a bikini wax?

There is no reason that you can't get waxed during pregnancy, but there are a couple of things to keep in mind. Many people report increased sensitivity during pregnancy, likely due to increased blood flow. You also may be uncomfortable lying on your back, but an experienced esthetician should be able to get you in and out quickly. Be sure to choose a clean and reputable salon to avoid the risk of infection.

Q. How much stress is too much stress?

Please try not to stress about being stressed. You have a lot going on, and a certain amount of stress and anxiety is expected. Everyone will tell you stress isn't good for the baby, which can cause you to be even more stressed out. Give yourself space to feel what you're feeling and reach out for help if needed. That being said, if you're going through extreme life changes or challenges and are concerned about the effects on your pregnancy, find help from a professional, and try various stress-reducing activities (see the following question). Between 7 and 25 percent of pregnant people suffer from depression during pregnancy; if you think this might be you, please talk to your provider right away.

Q. What are some ways to relieve stress during pregnancy?

There are a lot of small ways to reduce daily stress, and pregnancy is one of the best reasons ever to focus on you and your needs! First of all, make sure your basic needs are being met. Are you getting enough sleep? Eating a healthy diet? Getting in exercise when you can? Sleep, nutrition, and exercise can go a long way in reducing stress. Try getting some extra rest during the day if you can—even if you just close your eyes, a little "quiet wakefulness" can help with your mood and stress levels.

Next, think about what might be causing the stress and address or eliminate it from your life. Are you nervous about childbirth? Take a childbirth preparation class. Is there a friend or family member who is constantly upsetting you? It's okay to cut ties, at least through your pregnancy. Be up-front about how your interactions with them are causing you stress, or you can put the blame on your doctor or midwife by saying, "My doctor is concerned about my blood pressure and has asked me to reduce any stress, so I need to take some time and focus on staying well." If addressing the issue is too difficult, simply block their number and social media accounts until you're ready to reconnect.

Finally, find ways to practice self-care. Get a massage, make fun plans, diffuse essential oils, or add them to Epsom salts in your bath. You could also join a prenatal yoga class or start a meditation practice. Try Expectful, a guided meditation app specifically for expecting and new parents that focuses on helping you reduce stress, improve sleep, and connect with baby.

"I worked out as much as I could throughout both pregnancies, which definitely helped keep my energy up. An added bonus: I ended up having a C-section with my first son who was breech, and when the doctor opened me up, I heard him say, 'Wow, these are some nice abs.'"

—Lauren Goldsand Scarpati

7

Sex and Exercise

Lindsey Meehleis, LM, CPM

Are you wondering if you need to modify your exercise routine now that you're pregnant? Or maybe you or your partner are worried about how sex will affect your baby. Our midwife, Lindsey Meehleis, will cover all of your burning questions in this chapter so you can hopefully get on with your regularly scheduled activities.

Q. *Can my partner hurt the baby when we have sex?*

The short answer to this is no; however, if you have been put on pelvic rest, you will be advised to avoid sex. There is usually some sort of concern that your uterus shouldn't be stimulated by orgasm, or possibly you are told you have a short cervix or low-lying placenta and external stimulation could cause potential issues. If none of these apply to you, have fun! Your baby will be just fine and benefit from the oxytocin hormone release following sexual stimulation.

Q. *Are there any types of sex or sex positions I should abstain from while pregnant?*

Always see how you're feeling. Everyone has different anatomy, and while some positions might feel good to one person, they might feel awful to another. Be creative, especially as your belly grows in size. If it doesn't feel good, don't do it.

IF YOU'RE IN YOUR FIRST TRIMESTER

In the first trimester, usually all positions are comfortable because you don't have a large belly in the way. However, nausea and exhaustion can put a halt on one's sex life, and many people don't feel particularly sexy during this time. Talk to your partner, see what you're comfortable with, and communicate clearly what your needs are.

IF YOU'RE IN YOUR SECOND TRIMESTER

The second trimester is usually when your energy returns, you stop feeling bad, and your sex drive returns. While some people find a huge surge in their sex drive, others don't; both are normal. You might need to start getting creative with different sexual positions toward the end of the second trimester because the missionary position usually gets to be very awkward and uncomfortable. Plus, you shouldn't be lying on your back for an extended period of time.

IF YOU'RE IN YOUR THIRD TRIMESTER

In your third trimester, creativity is key. The sexual position that is most conducive to pleasure is sex from behind. However, this position can be very stimulating to the cervix, so if it doesn't feel good, try another position. The pregnant person being on top can also feel wonderful. Spooning, standing, oral sex, and anal sex are all things that you can try if you're curious. Allow yourself to unfold into all of this and learn how to pleasure yourself; remember, sex doesn't always require a partner. Go slowly, explore your sexuality in this new body, and welcome all things that come with this exploration.

Q. I noticed some light bleeding after sex. Is this normal?

The vagina is so vascular in pregnancy because of all of the extra blood volume, so bleeding from penetrative vaginal sex is not uncommon. While light bleeding and spotting are normal, heavy bleeding should be followed up with a call to your care provider to make sure all is well.

Q. I have zero sex drive. Is this normal?

This is very normal. You may not feel sexual at all during pregnancy. Your sex hormones depend on so many things, and while some feel like they want to have sex 24/7, others feel like they don't want to have sex at all. Listen to your body and consider exploring ways to be intimate with your partner that don't include sex.

Q. What are Kegel exercises, and should I be doing them? How do I do them?

Kegel exercises are the tightening of the pelvic-floor muscles, the same muscles that are contracted while trying to stop urination. The main reason that we talk of needing to exercise our pelvic floor is because humans have moved away from squatting throughout the day, a position that naturally engages this area. Strengthening your pelvic-floor muscles will help you better learn to control and relax them during labor, which can help you have an easier birth. To do a Kegel, start by identifying where the pelvic-floor muscles are by contracting them while you're peeing to stop the flow. Once you've figured that out, then pretend like you're taking these muscles on an elevator ride. Squeeze lightly at the first floor, more at the second floor, continuing to squeeze up to as tight as you can before slowly releasing your muscles back to the basement.

Q. What is pelvic-floor therapy, and do I need it?

Pelvic-floor therapy is a series of exercises that relax and strengthen the pelvic-floor muscles. In France, it's customary to receive this physical therapy for the first year after giving birth. If you see a pelvic-floor therapist during pregnancy, they will make individual recommendations based on what is best for you. Typically, they will give you suggested positions to push in during labor and exercises to release your pelvic floor for birth. Following birth, these therapists will do a vaginal exam to assess what your pelvic floor is doing and offer exercises and other treatment protocols to strengthen your pelvic floor. Talk to your midwife or OBGYN for a referral.

Q. Is it okay to exercise? What exercises are best? What exercises should I avoid?

Yes! Exercise is amazing and promotes wellness throughout pregnancy. The general recommendation is getting your heart rate up for more than 30 minutes, three to four times a week.

If you're an avid athlete, you can usually maintain the same workout schedule that your body is used to, but listen to your body. If it doesn't feel good, don't do it! If you want to start a new exercise regime during pregnancy, start slowly—this might not be the best time to train for a marathon. My favorite exercises are low-impact movement that gets your heart rate up, including walking, swimming, and yoga. These are exercises that anyone can do through all three trimesters.

High-impact exercises should be avoided if there are any concerns throughout your pregnancy. Birth Fit (BirthFit.com) is an organization that provides information about lifting weights during pregnancy. Discussing what you do with your care provider is what's most important because it's hard to make a general statement.

Q. I noticed some bleeding after exercising. Should I be concerned?

Your body has the unique capability to tell you when you're doing too much. This carries over into the postpartum period as well. If you notice spotting or bleeding, that typically means you're doing too much; take it down a few notches and listen to your body. If the bleeding is heavy or you have any concerns, contact your care provider.

"When I returned to work and had to leave my baby for the first time, I didn't know how I would possibly survive. I wanted to quit my job and cried at my desk for days. But, little by little, it got easier. Before I knew it, we're driving to daycare and my toddler is naming all of their friends at 'school,' and I realized how much love daycare has brought into their life, and how grateful I am for their second family."

—Liz Ekelund

8

Work and Taking Leave

Bryn Huntpalmer

Finding a balance between career and parenthood can be a never-ending struggle, and it isn't made any easier by our less-than-ideal parental leave policies in the United States. In this chapter we'll talk about how to navigate everything from sharing the news that you're pregnant with your supervisor to planning for maternity leave, finding childcare, and transitioning back to work. Find co-workers who have recently had babies and pick their brains about company policies, what worked well for them on leave, and for childcare recommendations.

Q. What's the best time to tell my employer that I'm expecting?

Most people wait until they start showing to tell their boss they're pregnant. However, if you're experiencing first trimester symptoms that are affecting your job performance and you feel comfortable sharing, let them know your news so they can accommodate you. Another time to let your employer know right away is if you work in an environment where you may be exposing the baby to toxins, like in a lab or around chemicals or radiation.

Q. How should I tell my boss I'm pregnant?

Schedule an in-person meeting and be straightforward and confident—you don't have anything to apologize for! Let them know when you're due, when you plan to start maternity leave, when you expect to return, and that you've already started working on a plan for covering your workload while you're out. It might be helpful to talk to a coworker who's recently had a baby or your human resources department to learn about your company's maternity leave policy so you can go into the meeting with as much information as possible.

Q. My job requires a lot of standing or heavy lifting. When should I stop these duties?

Heavy lifting, standing for long periods, and excessive bending have been associated with risks in pregnancy, including miscarriage and preterm labor. If you're lifting heavy objects, be sure to bend at the knees and push up with your legs rather than bending at the waist and straining your back. If your job requires any of these activities, talk to your care provider for tips on how to talk with your supervisor. Request the accommodations you need, especially after the first trimester. Keep in mind that you're protected by the U.S. Equal Employment Opportunity Commission. Find more information about pregnancy discrimination at eeoc.gov.

Q. *I sit at a desk all day. Is this bad for my baby?*

Sitting for long periods can lead to back pain and fluid retention. If you sit at a desk for most of the day, set an alarm on your phone to get up and move around every hour. It may also be a good idea to request accommodations like a standing desk or an exercise ball to sit on.

Q. *What is FMLA, and what do I need to know about it?*

The Family and Medical Leave Act (FMLA), is a law enforced by the U.S. Department of Labor regarding time off from work for family and medical reasons. FMLA requires all public agencies and private companies with more than 50 employees to allow up to 12 weeks of unpaid leave for a serious health condition, and giving birth falls under this umbrella. Consult with human resources about your options around extended leave and the use of FMLA. You must request FMLA at least 30 days before taking it. You can find more information on the Department of Labor website at dol.gov.

Q. *I know each state is different when it comes to parental leave. Where do I find out information about my state?*

Unfortunately, as of the writing of this book, the majority of states do not provide any protection for parents beyond what is required by FMLA, which is 12 weeks of unpaid leave. Some states offer an additional layer of job protection but no paid benefits, and the laws are often vague and open to employer interpretation. However, there are a few states leading the way in making positive changes in this area. California, Connecticut, Hawaii, Massachusetts, New Jersey, New York, Rhode Island, Washington, and the District of Columbia have all implemented or passed laws requiring paid benefits for parental leave. You can read about these policies at policygenius.com/blog/parental-leave-by-state.

Additionally, some companies are taking the lead on parental leave and have their own generous policies in place. Look into the parental leave policies of individual employers if you or your partner are considering job changes in the near future.

Q. How long should I take for parental leave?

Unfortunately, the United States has one of the worst parental leave policies, or lack thereof, in the world. Many European countries offer a year or more of leave for both parents. I bring this up to draw attention to the fact that our perception of how long new parents should take off from work is greatly skewed by what we have come to accept as normal in the United States. Research shows that the optimal amount of time for parental leave is one year of paid leave split between two parents. But that isn't going to be most people's reality in the United States.

The amount of leave you take is going to vary widely for each individual, so take as long as your family and job situation allow. Most first-time parents are surprised by the physical and mental toll that new parenthood takes on them. The more time you have to recover from birth and bond with your baby, the better. Look at your finances, talk to your partner if you have one, and discuss your options with your supervisor. See if you can start part-time and work your way back up to full-time over the span of a few weeks or months.

If you're self-employed, try to plan ahead and find help, even if it's temporary, so that you can unplug for a bit after the baby arrives.

Q. How should I prepare for parental leave?

By the middle of your third trimester, begin working on your parental leave plans. If you work for a company, schedule a meeting with your team and discuss how your work will be handled in your absence. If you work for yourself, try to frontload your work so you can unplug for at least a few weeks. Set an out-of-office response in your email that you can activate when the time comes. Look for new parent meet-ups and support groups so that you're getting out of the house and socializing once you feel up for it during your leave. Staying home with baby can feel isolating when you're used to being surrounded by other adults all day.

Q. How can I prepare for returning to work from parental leave?

Check in with your supervisor a couple of weeks before you plan to return to work to see if you can adjust your schedule as needed. This is also a good time to make sure there is a place to pump if you're breastfeeding and plan to continue doing so from work. If you plan to work from home, you likely still need help. Newborns are unpredictable, so it's hard to schedule work around their naps, or lack thereof. Try to find at least a few hours of childcare for each day.

Q. What do I need to know about finding childcare?

If you're planning to return to work, start looking into childcare options before baby arrives because in some areas, daycares fill up fast; nannies are often planning ahead when moving from one family to the next. Ask friends for recommendations, schedule tours of daycare centers, or find a nanny agency so you can get on any waiting lists.

If you know you will have childcare expenses, look into a dependent care FSA with your employer or your partner's employer. This is where your company can take pretax money from your paycheck and put it into an account that you can pull from to cover childcare expenses. It can save you about 30 percent on childcare. If your employers don't offer this, you should still keep your childcare receipts because you can take advantage of the Child and Dependent Care Credit when you file your tax return.

"I know now that I'm a turbo-nester. In my first and second pregnancies I didn't allow time for preparing my home for baby. Then, before my third and fourth, I nested in manic glory and had magical births and postpartum. For me, nesting is the most important preparation for birth."

—Tess Noren

CHAPTER

9

Preparing for Baby

Bryn Huntpalmer

There are many things you *can* do when preparing for baby, but there's really not a ton that you *must* do! Despite all of the advertisements and adorable Instagram shops inundating your feed, babies don't need a lot when they're itty-bitty. We will go over the preparation basics in this chapter so you feel prepared but hopefully not overwhelmed as you wait for your little one's arrival.

Q. What are the must-do tasks before baby arrives?

» Get necessities for baby (see the following question).
» Interview and choose a pediatrician.
» Take a baby care class, including infant CPR.
» Get your infant car seat installed and have it checked by a cer-
  tified Child Passenger Safety Technician (CPST). You can find
  one at safekids.org.
» Prepare a safe place for your baby to sleep.
» Order a free breast pump through insurance using a service like
  aeroflowbreastpumps.com.

Q. What should I register for?

Most baby registries are online now, so you don't even have to get out
of your pajamas. Babylist is a universal, online registry that allows
you to pull items from any store. Babylist also offers up-to-date shopping guides and sample registries. There are hundreds of different
options for each category and tons of items that either are irresistibly
cute or will make your life easier.

BABY REGISTRY BASICS

» Car seat
» Diapers and wipes
» 10 outfits (infant gowns, sleepers, or onesies and baby hats
  depending on the season)
» 10 burp cloths (I like using cloth diaper prefolds for this)
» Safe place for baby to sleep
» Swaddles
» Pacifier (register for a few different types to see what your
  baby prefers)
» A safe, convenient place to put your baby while you take
  a shower or use the bathroom, like a baby seat or
  portable bassinet

- » A front baby carrier, wrap, or sling
- » Baby care: thermometer, baby nail clippers or file, snot sucker (I like the NoseFrida)
- » If bottle feeding: formula, bottles, bottle brush
- » If breastfeeding: nursing bra, breast pads, breast pump, nipple cream

Q. How do I prepare my budget for a baby?

It's never too early to start looking at your finances and making a plan for things like paying for prenatal care and childcare once baby arrives. Call your health insurance company for an estimate of out-of-pocket expenses for prenatal care and birth. Next, sit down with your partner, if you have one, and take stock of your monthly income and expenses. Then calculate how your income may change during maternity leave, and plan for additional baby-related expenses. A 2010 USDA report showed that the average middle-income family spent around $12,000 on child-related expenses in their baby's first year of life. Make plans to cut back on unnecessary expenses if needed.

Q. What is cord blood banking, and should I do it?

Cord blood banking is when stem cells from your baby's umbilical cord blood are preserved and stored in a blood bank. These stem cells can be used to treat leukemia and other life-threatening diseases should your baby or a future sibling need them. If you decide to look into this, there are several companies that offer this service, so you should get a few cost breakdowns. Many hospitals also offer the option to donate cord blood that could be used to save another life. Find out more at bethematch.org.

Q. What do I need to know about circumcision?

Circumcision is a surgical procedure to remove your baby's fore-skin, which is a sheath of skin surrounding the tip, or glans, of the penis. This can be a heated topic in the United States. It used to be common to circumcise, but there's been a significant decline in recent years—a 2009 survey showed that only about 50 percent of baby boys are circumcised, and it's likely that even fewer babies are being circumcised today.

Some parents make the decision to circumcise for religious reasons or based on whether the baby's father is circumcised. Many parents want to know if circumcision causes pain, if it is medically necessary, if it affects sexual intimacy, etc. I encourage you to do your own research. The most comprehensive, evidence-based, and unbiased resource online regarding circumcision can be found at evidencebasedbirth.com/circumcisionfaqs/.

Q. What's a doula, and do I need one?

A birth doula is someone trained to provide emotional, physical, and informational support throughout your labor. A postpartum doula comes to your house to help take care of you and baby during the day or overnight and help with household tasks. Studies have shown that mothers who have a doula at their birth have lower rates of epidurals, cesareans, use of Pitocin (synthetic oxytocin, which induces con-tractions), and the use of forceps or vacuum assistance. Larger cities will host gatherings where expecting parents can meet with a bunch of doulas in the area, kind of like speed dating. If you don't have an event like this in your city, try DoulaMatch.net or Dona.org. If you're on a tight budget, some hospitals have volunteer doula programs, or you may be able to find a doula-in-training who will waive their fee.

Q. I keep hearing I should take a childbirth class. What are my options?

There are several options for childbirth classes as well as laboring methods.

HOSPITAL BIRTH CLASSES

Hospital birth classes are usually focused on learning the practices/policies of your hospital or practice and how to be a good patient. If you feel confident that your hospital or care provider has your best interests in mind, then these classes are a great way to know what to expect at your particular birthing location. Another advantage is that the cost tends to be lower than an independent class or even free, since this class is supported by the hospital or practice. Keep in mind that these classes are often limited by the policies and preferences of the hospital and may not give you a full picture of all of your birthing options. Take the hospital class if it's free or low cost so you can get an idea of what they expect your birth to look like, and then seek an independently taught class as well for more comprehensive childbirth education.

ONLINE CHILDBIRTH CLASSES

If you're having trouble finding time in your schedule or if the idea of learning about placentas in a room full of strangers doesn't sound appealing to you, you also have the option to take an online childbirth class. Through my work with *The Birth Hour*, I found that many birthgivers were looking for a childbirth course that wasn't only tailored to unmedicated births, so we created an evidence-based course called "Know Your Options" that addresses all types of childbirth methods—unmedicated, epidurals, C-sections, and more. This course takes you all the way through postpartum, breastfeeding, and even going back to work after baby. You can find this course at TheBirthHour.com.

THE BRADLEY METHOD

The Bradley Method focuses on the partner taking a very active role in helping the birthing parent stay relaxed and thus able to cope with the intensity of labor. These classes often help parents achieve a low-intervention, unmedicated birth. Bradley Method classes are taught in person and are 12 weeks long.

HYPNOBIRTHING AND HYPNOBABIES

HypnoBirthing® and Hypnobabies® both use guided relaxation scripts and self-hypnosis techniques to cope with labor. HypnoBirthing has been around longer, there are more instructors out there teaching in-person classes, and you can also buy a HypnoBirthing book to read on your own. Hypnobabies is a newer technique, so it may be more difficult to find an instructor, but they do offer a home-study course.

LAMAZE

Lamaze has been around since 1960 and used to be known primarily for its breathing techniques. Lamaze has updated its curriculum, has dropped the emphasis on learning specific breathing techniques, and now focuses on helping parents have a safe and healthy birth through teaching "Six Healthy Birth Practices." Lamaze instructors can be found teaching both in hospitals and independently.

BIRTHING FROM WITHIN

Birthing from Within refers to partners as "birth guardians or loving partners" rather than coaches. Birthing from Within sees birth as a rite of passage or "heroic journey," which, regardless of birth outcome, can be an occasion to practice awareness. Birthing from Within instructors view themselves as mentors, guiding you in self-discovery and working through fears.

Q. Should I have a birth plan? If so, what should it include?

You will hear mixed responses from birth professionals when it comes to writing a birth plan. In *The Birth Hour*'s "Know Your Options" childbirth course, we refer to creating a list of "birth preferences" because the fact of the matter is that birth is unpredictable. It's smart to know your options and consider what you want, but keep in mind that it may not go according to plan, and your preferences may change as labor progresses. Some things to consider are:

» Who do you want in the labor room with you? Are you okay with medical students or residents in your labor room?

» Do you want pain relief discussed right away or only if you ask for it?

» Do you want to walk around and move in labor?

» Do you want to self-hydrate (with a saline lock in case IV hydration is needed)?

» Do you want to limit the number of cervical exams, or would you like to be checked at regular intervals?

» How do you feel about having your water broken to augment labor?

» Do you want to be offered various positions to push in? Do you want a mirror while pushing? Do you want the option of using a squat bar? Do you want to use the stirrups?

» Do you want coaching or counting while pushing, or do you prefer to push instinctively?

» Do you want perineal massage or warm compresses while pushing?

» Do you want immediate skin to skin or for baby to be cleaned and swaddled first? Do you want to delay newborn care procedures like weighing and measuring until after your first experience of bonding or breastfeeding?

» Do you want delayed cord clamping, if possible? Whom do you want to cut the cord?

» Do you want visitors in labor and delivery, or do you want them to wait until you're moved to your postpartum room?

» Do you plan to exclusively breastfeed in the hospital, feed the baby formula, or a combination?

» Would you like a lactation consultant to come by on day one or wait until you ask for support?

» Do you want to keep your baby with you, or would you like baby to go to the nursery so you can rest?

» If the baby needs to be taken somewhere for a procedure, would you (or your partner) like to go with your baby?

» Do you plan to circumcise your baby?

» Do you want the standard newborn treatments, like erythromycin eye ointment, vitamin K injection, or the hepatitis B vaccination? You can decline these things but will likely need to sign a waiver.

Q. Are there any classes I should take on breastfeeding and baby care?

Some childbirth classes, including *The Birth Hour*'s "Know Your Options" online course, will cover newborn care as well. If yours does not, I recommend finding a baby care class that also includes instruction on infant CPR (you can find one at RedCross.org). If you plan to breastfeed, consider finding a breastfeeding class or a support group (like La Leche League) or meeting with a lactation consultant prior to your baby's arrival.

Q. Should I hire a birth photographer? How do I find one?

The day you give birth is also the day you meet your baby and your heart expands more than you ever thought possible. It's also likely one of the hardest days of your life as your body goes through the challenging process of giving birth. For many people, it's a bit of a blur, and having someone there to document it can be an incredible gift. Birth photographers are familiar with the birth process, so they know how to navigate a labor room and can make themselves barely noticeable. You can find one by asking for recommendations from doulas or other birth professionals in your area or looking on BirthBecomesHer.com.

Q. What are some things I can do to prepare for postpartum?

Create a list of action items for your family and friends to help with after baby arrives. Some ideas include dog walking, meal prep, laundry, house cleaning, and grocery shopping. You can also do some prep ahead of time like stocking up on freezer meals.

Gathering supplies for your postpartum recovery is one of the best things you can do to make those first few weeks go more smoothly. A lot of what you will need postpartum depends on how your birth goes and whether you run into any breastfeeding issues. We'll cover more on postpartum care supplies in Chapter 11 (page 131) and breastfeeding supplies in Chapter 12 (page 149).

"One of the hardest, but most important, elements of childbirth is trusting your body. After I stopped dilating at 8 centimeters with my first, I had a lot of distrust with my body and medicated birth. I think interventions are there for amazing reasons but get overused on new moms. I think we need to trust our bodies and get more comfortable with the idea of being uncomfortable—that not all pain is bad. Sometimes we need to lean into it."

—Caitlin Shrum

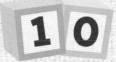

Labor and Childbirth

Lindsey Meehleis, LM, CPM and
Dr. Emiliano Chavira, MD, MPH, FACOG

Preparing for your baby to make its appearance is likely at the forefront of your mind, and if this is your first pregnancy, you probably have a lot of questions. This chapter is divided between our midwife and OBGYN experts and will cover all things labor: signs, stages, coping, progression, and potential interventions. We'll also cover labor preferences and what's typical of most hospitals when it comes to things like epidurals, cesarean births, and NICU stays. Because birth is unpredictable, this is one chapter where we recommend reading through all of the questions in case the unexpected occurs.

Q. What is a Braxton-Hicks contraction?

A Braxton-Hicks contraction is the tightening of the uterus to tone the muscle in preparation for birth. These are normal and can occur from the beginning of pregnancy until birth. Typically, during your first pregnancy, you may not recognize the sensation until your uterus gets larger, but for someone who has had more than one baby, they're more easily noticed. They feel like the tightening of the belly or the contraction of a muscle, like when you're lifting weights. Some people notice them more if they are walking, exercising, or dehydrated. If you note more than six in an hour and they are getting closer and stronger in consistency or if you have any other questions or concerns, contact your care provider.

Q. What is prodromal labor or "false labor"?

Prodromal labor, or false labor, is contractions that don't promote cervical dilation. These contractions can be close together and painful and cause you to miss sleep. They can also be extremely discouraging because you don't feel like you're working toward a goal (birth). It's more common for people who have had more than one baby to experience this, and it can last for weeks. Prodromal labor is also common with a mispositioned baby (e.g., posterior). In this situation, you can try some Spinning Babies exercises (SpinningBabies.com) to get your baby into the optimal fetal position. This typically resets labor and will either stop prodromal labor contractions or will make them more effective, leading to active labor.

Q. I keep reading that there are foods or teas that can induce labor. Do any of them actually work? What about herbal supplements or essential oils?

If you look on the Internet, there is a mile-long list of all the things you can do to try to get your baby to come, from having sex and bouncing on birth balls to eating pineapple and drinking red raspberry leaf tea. There are even restaurants that sell famed "labor induction" dishes with lines out the door!

One of the most common methods people have reported trying is taking evening primrose oil orally or vaginally. However, there is almost no research on the efficacy of evening primrose oil in inducing labor. One randomized trial found evening primrose oil did improve cervical ripening, but it made no difference in how quickly labor began. Another study found a trend toward labor complications in the group that took evening primrose oil. In reality, unless your baby is truly ready, these methods typically don't help induce labor— even if a friend, or a friend of a friend, reported success with one.

There are "natural" methods of induction, like using blue and black cohosh herbs or castor oil to help contract your uterus. However, both of these are actually quite aggressive methods and are not recommended to use by yourself. Cohosh can be dangerous, and castor oil, when taken in high doses, is a strong laxative, causing diarrhea, which irritates your uterus into contracting.

It's understandable that you're feeling impatient about meeting your baby or are simply just tired of being pregnant. But remember that there is an increased risk with any form of intervention, including induction, so it's recommended that you consult with your care provider to see if your baby is ready or if there is a medical need for induction before trying any of these methods.

Q. Can things like acupressure/acupuncture and massage help induce labor?

Practitioners of Traditional Chinese Medicine (TCM) stimulate specific points along the meridians, or pathways through which chi (energy) flows, to help with the induction of labor. Many TCM practitioners recommend starting these treatments around week 37 of pregnancy as a way to prepare the body for birth. Evidence Based Birth has created a wonderful video that explains using acupuncture to induce labor (evidencebasedbirth.com/evidence-acupuncture-to -induce-labor/).

Q. What is a membrane sweep, and should I get one to induce labor?

A membrane sweep is when your practitioner inserts their finger into your vagina and through your cervix, if it is open enough, to run their finger along the rim of your cervix where the amniotic sac is attached, attempting to "detach" it from your cervix and stir up a "hormonal cocktail," if you will, to get labor moving. Just by irritating the cervix and encouraging more dilation, a membrane sweep can cause your uterus to contract and help induce labor.

A membrane sweep doesn't come without risk and can cause a premature artificial rupture of your membranes (water breaking). If you tested positive for group B strep (GBS), a membrane sweep can increase your baby's risk of infection because a manual exam brings the bacteria further up into your cervix. Also, membrane sweeps aren't the most comfortable procedures, and they can be especially uncomfortable for you if you have any history of sexual abuse, so be open with your care provider and advocate for what you feel is appropriate for your body.

Q. Are there any risks of inducing labor?

Induction of labor does have risks, so it's best to avoid induction unless there is an appropriate reason to do so. If your labor is induced, you will likely be on the labor and delivery ward for several hours longer than if you walk into the hospital in spontaneous labor. More time may also mean more cervical exams, and both time and cervical exams can increase the chances of developing a fever or infection in labor. Medications that cause the uterus to contract (like prostaglandins and oxytocin) can overstimulate the uterus and cause contractions that are stronger and closer together. In some cases, this could even potentially affect the baby by reducing the blood and oxygen flow to the placenta. This is why a medical induction should be done carefully and only when medically indicated. Protocols should be followed, and fetal monitoring should be done to make sure that the uterus is not being overstimulated and that the baby is tolerating the induction well.

Q. What indicators are there that an induction will work?

If the cervix is already soft and a few centimeters dilated, the induction is more likely to lead to vaginal birth than if the cervix is long and closed. If you have had a vaginal birth already in a prior pregnancy, you're more likely to have a successful induction than someone who has never given birth vaginally before. Also, the further along in your pregnancy you are, the more likely it is that the induction will lead to a vaginal birth. The earlier you are in your pregnancy, the higher the chances that the induction might not work and you end up with a cesarean birth.

In order to determine whether you're a good candidate for induction, your provider can perform a vaginal exam and give you a Bishop score, based on a pre-labor scoring system that involves looking at your cervical positioning, the consistency of your cervix, your cervical effacement and dilation, and where your baby is within your pelvis to determine whether induction will be successful for you. These things combined will give you a number, and the closer you are to a 13, the more likely induction will work.

However, the likelihood of success should not be the reason to induce or not induce labor. The main reason to induce labor is if you're in a situation where it is thought to be safer to bring the baby out into the world than to continue the pregnancy.

Q. What are the medical methods for inducing labor?

If the cervix is still long and closed, there will usually be a period of "cervical ripening" before starting the actual induction. Cervical ripening involves the use of either a mechanical device or a medication to cause the cervix to soften up and dilate, usually up to three or four centimeters. Cervical ripening varies in how long it takes, but on average it takes about 12 hours. Methods include the following:

Cervical balloon. For this method, a soft flexible catheter with a small balloon at the end is inserted into the cervix. The balloon is inflated to about the size of a lime. The catheter may be taped to your leg to provide tension.

Mechanical dilators. For this method, several thin sticks about the size of a match are inserted into the cervix. These sticks absorb liquid, so they expand slowly over the next few hours, causing the cervix to soften and dilate a few centimeters.

Prostaglandins. Prostaglandins are hormones that are already naturally involved in the labor process. They can be delivered via a gel, pills, or a little plastic insert on a string.

If the cervix is already soft and a few centimeters dilated, you will skip all cervical ripening methods and go straight to the induction of labor. Sometimes the cervical ripening method itself can start labor, and additional induction methods may not be required. Some induction methods include the following:

Oxytocin (Pitocin). This is the main and most common method for a medical induction of labor. Oxytocin is given through an IV, starting at a low dose and increasing gradually until a regular contraction pattern is obtained. An oxytocin induction may take 12 to 24 hours on average.

Rupture of membranes. This method involves using a plastic hook to break the bag of water. At term, this may trigger labor. Rupturing membranes as the sole method of inducing labor is used less often than other methods. However, rupturing membranes *during* an ongoing induction to help speed things along is very common.

Castor oil. This method involves drinking a solution with castor oil in it for a laxative effect, which stimulates labor. This method has fewer studies behind it compared to other methods. Midwives are more likely to use castor oil than doctors. This method can also be used without going to the hospital, whereas other methods of induction are done only in a hospital setting.

Q. What are the most common reasons for an induction?

Induction of labor is done when it is thought to be safer to deliver the baby than to continue the pregnancy. Some common examples include post-term pregnancy, low amniotic fluid in a term pregnancy, preeclampsia, growth restriction (poor fetal growth), or some significant medical complications such as diabetes, hypertension, lupus, or kidney disease. If you're having antepartum testing done (see the section on NSTs, page 31, for more information on antepartum testing), an abnormal test of fetal well-being might be a reason to induce labor.

Q. Are dilation and effacement indicators of when I will go into labor?

The status of the cervix when you're full term doesn't accurately predict when labor will begin. Some really want to know when labor is going to happen, but, unfortunately, there is no real way to know that with certainty. Your cervix may be closed, and you might still go into labor within a day or two of that cervical exam. Alternatively, your cervix might be soft and a few centimeters dilated, but it could still be a few weeks before you go into labor. Although people love to predict when labor will begin (including pregnancy care professionals), the reality is that no one can know for sure.

Q. Did I pee myself, or did my water break? How will I know?

It can be hard to tell. In some cases, the water breaks, a large gush of fluid flows out, and it's obvious what has happened. In other cases, only a small leak occurs. When the leak is small, it can be hard to tell if it's amniotic fluid, vaginal discharge, sperm from recent intercourse, or even sweat. There is no real way for you to tell the difference. If you have any new leakage of fluid from the vagina, you will need to be examined. There are a few tests that your care provider can do to determine whether your water has broken.

Q. What would be a good reason for having my water broken? What are the risks?

Having your water broken, or what is known as artificial rupture of membranes, is considered a full-fledged method of induction and is more typically done in hospital settings. Artificially breaking a person's bag of waters is done because it is thought to speed up the start of labor or because your care provider needs to monitor the well-being of the baby. Once your bag of waters is broken, you're considered in labor and immediately put on a time clock. In the 1950s and 1960s, care providers routinely performed cesareans after 24 hours of labor. Current research doesn't support this, but it is still a practice in some hospitals. While studies indicate that between 77 and 95 percent of people will go into labor within 24 hours of their water breaking, these statistics are based on your bag of water breaking on its own. One potential risk of having your water broken artificially is the increased possibility of needing further intervention like a C-section. Another main risk of this intervention is the increased risk of infection, especially if you tested positive for group B strep. Talk to your provider and know what their recommendations are if you don't start labor within 24 hours of having your water broken. Weigh the benefits, risks, and alternatives, and see what option suits you best.

Q. My water broke, but I'm not having contractions. What should I do?

First things first, check for the following important things: the color and smell of the fluid and baby's movements. If the color is not clear, if the fluid smells foul, or if the baby doesn't seem to be moving normally, then call your provider immediately. However, if the fluid is clear, there is no foul smell, and baby is moving normally, then all of this is within normal limits. You should still call and have a discussion with your care provider because each practitioner will have a different policy. Many OBs, because of hospital liability, will send you straight to the hospital for monitoring, while many midwives will provide instructions for monitoring and mitigating infection, like taking your temperature and using immune-boosting supplements like vitamin C—and, if it's the middle of the night, send you back to bed to get some much-needed sleep until the action picks up.

Q. Are there any restrictions once my water is broken?

This will really depend on how many weeks along you are, the position of the baby, the preferences of your care provider, and whether you're planning a home or hospital birth. If your water breaks and you're still preterm (less than 37 weeks), you will probably be instructed to head straight to the hospital. If you're past 37 weeks and the baby is in a head-down position, the water breaking is usually not an emergency situation. Some providers may want you to come to the hospital right away. Others may recommend that you wait for uterine contractions to begin as long as the baby is moving well, there is no fever, and the fluid is clear. You will need to get specific advice from your care provider for your specific situation and birth plan. After your water breaks, you can minimize the risk of infection to both you and baby by not having intercourse, making sure you are wiping from front to back during trips to the bathroom, limiting cervical exams, and staying out of bodies of water that are open to the public, like a shared tub, Jacuzzi, or pool.

Q. How will I know if my contractions are the real deal?

If you're questioning whether the contractions you're feeling are the real deal, chances are they're probably not. Typically, there's no questioning real contractions, unless you have some serious pain tolerance! What we're looking for are contractions that are getting longer, stronger, and closer together. Active labor is typically when contractions are three to four minutes apart and lasting 60 seconds and you can't talk through them. Labor contractions are sometimes associated with "bloody show," a thick vaginal discharge made up of mucus and blood. The purpose of uterine contractions is to push the baby lower into your pelvis and also to help dilate your cervix by pulling up on both sides, shortening and opening it. Your baby works with every contraction to tuck and rotate through your pelvis.

Q. When should I go to the hospital or birth center?

Ideally you want to avoid arriving at the hospital too early, which sometimes leads to unnecessary interventions. It's best to arrive when you're already in active labor (usually six centimeters dilated or more). It's hard to judge this without a cervical exam, especially if this is your first labor. A general rule of thumb is that if you're having strong contractions that make you breathe hard every five minutes or so for an hour or two without letting up, there is a good chance you're in active labor. If you start to see vaginal bleeding, this can also be a sign of active labor. You might head out sooner if you have a long drive ahead of you, so use your judgment. Also, if you have had vaginal births in the past, this labor may go faster. The more babies you have had, the faster labor tends to be, so adjust accordingly. Again, contractions every five minutes for one to two hours is a general guideline. If you have not met those exact criteria but feel the pain is getting too intense to tolerate, you may decide to head in earlier.

Q. I'm having a home birth. When should I call the midwife?

Every midwife has different guidelines regarding when they want you to call based on how many babies you have had, how far they live from you, etc. Be sure to discuss this with your midwife. In my own practice, with first-time birthgivers, I like them to be in a very active labor phase. I find that if I come too early, contractions slow and they essentially become like a watched pot. I tell my patients that they should have me come when they think they need to be doing something different because they can't handle the intensity anymore. With my clients who have had more than one baby, I don't have a rule per se; I ask them to trust their bodies and tell me when they think they need me, but typically I come when contractions are around four to five minutes apart.

Q. Will I be able to eat and drink during labor?

Historically, hospitals have been very strict about not permitting eating or drinking during labor. This was based on the concern that you might vomit during an emergency cesarean and aspirate some of that fluid into your lungs. This is very rare but can be very serious. In recent years, there has been research that supports the safety of light eating and drinking during labor. Some labor and delivery units are starting to loosen their restrictions on food and drink intake during labor, especially clear fluids. Some hospitals, though, still have those old-fashioned policies of no eating or drinking in labor. If you're planning a birth-center birth or a home birth, you're more likely to have freedom to move, eat, and drink at will, although once in active labor, you likely won't have much of an appetite.

Q. Do I have to get an IV at the hospital?

At a hospital, an IV is placed as a routine measure, as IV fluids are usually given during labor. Routine medications such as pain medication or antibiotics can also be given through IV if needed. If uterine contractions slow down or space out, IV oxytocin (Pitocin) can be given to keep the labor moving along. The IV also serves as a safety precaution. If an emergency comes up suddenly, it can be used to quickly give fluids, emergency medications, or even a blood transfusion if necessary. Technically, you have the right to say no to the IV. You have the right to say no to any intervention or treatment that you're not willing to receive. However, the reality is that while many care providers will be open to discussing your preferences and will ultimately respect your wishes, there are some providers who may aggressively try to push or even force you to follow their policies and procedures. To avoid getting into a serious argument with your care providers while you're in labor, it's wise to discuss the details of your birth ahead of time. If you give birth at home or a freestanding birth center, an IV is usually not placed as a matter of routine but may be placed to give fluids or medications if the need arises.

Q. What is the difference between intermittent and continuous monitoring?

Fetal monitoring involves attaching a small ultrasound device to your belly to monitor your baby's heartbeat during labor. The theory behind this practice is that you might be able to detect cases where the baby is getting into trouble, and then you can deliver quickly to prevent brain injury during the childbirth process. With continuous monitoring, the ultrasound device is left attached to you at all times, and the goal is to listen to the baby's heartbeat nonstop until the birth. Intermittent monitoring means that the baby's heartbeat is monitored for a short period like 20 minutes, repeated every so often, like every two hours. Studies of fetal monitoring have not clearly shown that either method actually prevents cases of brain damage in the baby. On the other hand, it does appear that fetal monitoring increases the chances of an operative vaginal birth or a cesarean. Despite the fact that the benefit of fetal monitoring is unclear, continuous electronic fetal monitoring is a routine practice in labor and delivery units. Some units do have intermittent monitoring protocols. If you give birth at home or in a birth center, fetal monitoring is usually intermittent.

Q. What pain medications are available at the hospital?

There are three main pain medication options available:

An epidural. This is a catheter that is inserted into your back, almost like an IV line. The pain medication drips through that line slowly, numbing the nerves going to your uterus and pelvis. It is usually very effective at reducing pain. See the following question for more on epidurals.

Nitrous oxide. This is a gas given via a face mask that you breathe through. It can relieve anxiety and reduce labor pain. It is common in Canada, the United Kingdom, and Scandinavia and less commonly used in the United States, but some American hospitals may have it. Some birth centers may have it as well. It does not appear to have any harmful effects on the baby but can cause drowsiness, dizziness, or nausea in the mother. The effects of nitrous oxide wear off within a few minutes once you stop breathing through the mask.

Narcotics, also known as opioids. These are medications like morphine and fentanyl. They are given through the IV, although morphine can also be given as an injection into a muscle. These medications take effect right away and last for an hour or two before wearing off. They don't eliminate labor pain completely but may make it more bearable. They can cause drowsiness or dizziness and sometimes nausea. Opioids do enter the baby's bloodstream and can cause drowsiness and reduced breathing in the baby, which is not a problem during labor. However, it can become a problem when the baby is born. Because of this, opioids are usually avoided if the delivery is expected to happen soon so that the baby is not born with those side effects.

Q. What are the pros and cons of getting an epidural?

An epidural is probably the most effective method for pain control in labor. Most of the time the epidural works so well that you can't even feel the contractions anymore. As well as epidurals work while the cervix is dilating, it is common to feel some pressure again or even pain during the actual childbirth itself, so don't expect an epidural to make childbirth completely painless. Another benefit is that an epidural can last for as long as the labor lasts (as opposed to IV pain medications, which will wear off after an hour or two). If you end up having a cesarean, the epidural can be used for the surgery. If you're planning to have your tubes tied after the birth, the same epidural can often be used for that procedure as well.

There are some downsides to an epidural. The epidural catheter has to be inserted into your back, so it is an additional procedure. It takes about half an hour or so for the anesthesiologist to take your history, set up all the materials, and insert and test the epidural. While you're likely to feel much less pain when the epidural is activated, your legs are also likely to feel numb and heavy. For some this is a very unsettling feeling, but it will wear off over time. You will also need a catheter to relieve urine and won't be able to get up and walk around while the epidural is in place or for a while after birth. An epidural can also slow down labor to some degree. Epidurals are very safe, but some complications can occur. About 2 percent of the time an epidural may not work very well. There is also a small chance that it may decrease your blood pressure, creating a problem for the baby. Usually the problem can be corrected by changing your position, giving IV fluids, and possibly even giving a medication to raise the blood pressure back up to a normal level. In rare cases, if your blood pressure doesn't improve, this can be a reason for an emergency C-section. In about 1 percent of cases, the epidural can cause a bad headache for a few days after the birth. Some people worry about complications like nerve damage or paralysis. While there have been cases of things like this happening, they are extremely rare and not worth worrying about.

Q. What is a walking epidural?

A walking epidural involves the placement of an epidural catheter into the same location in your back, but the medications are given in lower doses. The goal is to provide some pain relief without numbing the legs so that you can still stand or even walk. Because lower doses are used, the pain control may not be the same as when full doses are used.

Q. Will my partner/doula be able to stay with me at all times?

Usually the visiting hours on labor and delivery units are 24/7. Your support team should be able to stay with you throughout labor and the birth, although some units place a limit on how many people can be in the labor room with you at any one time. If you have a cesarean with an epidural or spinal (a one-time injection in the back that numbs the lower half of your body), typically one support person is allowed into the OR with you. You're welcome to ask if more than one person might be allowed in. If you have a cesarean under general anesthesia (when you're put to sleep completely), then no one will be allowed into the OR during the surgery. After the birth, you will likely be moved to a postpartum ward for one to three days. These units typically have specified visiting hours. If the postpartum rooms are private, your partner or other support person will probably be permitted to stay with you overnight. If the rooms are shared, you may not be able to have visitors overnight. You can get detailed answers to these specific questions on the hospital tour.

Q. What are the stages of labor?

There are four stages of labor:

EARLY LABOR, ACTIVE LABOR, AND TRANSITION
The first stage includes three phases: The first is early labor, which typically involves the thinning of the cervix with dilation to around four to five centimeters. During this time, contractions are likely mild to moderate and more spaced apart. They may not even have a regular pattern. It's an exciting time, but it's important to relax and preserve your energy now—you'll need it later! The next phase is called active labor, which begins when you are about six centimeters dilated. Contractions are more regular and intense. The third phase is

called transition, or "transformation," as many midwives prefer to call it. This is when you are fully dilated (or close to it), and it is typically the shortest yet most intense stage of labor. This stage can last for 15 minutes or for several hours. Contractions are very close together and strong, and you usually feel great pressure on your lower back and rectum and an urge to push. At this point, it's very common to feel like you can't keep going and you can't labor any longer. Lean on your support team and let them know exactly what you need from them. You are capable; let them help you through it.

THE PUSHING STAGE

The second stage of labor is when you move into the pushing phase. In a physiological birth, which is a birth with no interventions, this pushing usually happens uncontrollably because the baby puts pressure on the rectal nerves—this feels a lot like when you have to poop. With an epidural, this urge to push is typically numbed, so the pushing might look a little different and more directed. Your care provider may perform a cervical check and ask you to begin pushing once you are fully dilated. The goal is to push with each contraction so you are working with your contracting uterus to push the baby out. This stage of labor lasts until the baby is born.

AFTERBIRTH

The third stage of labor is the time from after the baby is born until the birth of the placenta. If the placenta is born physiologically— again, without intervention—it typically comes out anywhere from 10 minutes to 90 minutes after the baby. In a hospital setting, the placenta is delivered around 30 minutes after the baby as they actively manage the third stage of labor. In some midwifery practices, the birth of the placenta happens on its own as long as bleeding is under control.

RECOVERY

The fourth stage of labor is the recovery following the birth of your baby. While there is no true time frame for how long this stage lasts, as mentioned elsewhere in this book, many consider this the fourth trimester and treat it like a regular trimester that lasts 12 weeks. This is a time for your body to recover from pregnancy and birth while you're also learning to feed and take care of your baby. A nice rule of thumb at the beginning of this time is five days in bed, five days around the bed and bedroom, and five days around the house. Slowly ease yourself back into your routines and remember that this time will go by quickly, so enjoy it as much as you can.

Q. What are some coping strategies I can use to manage labor pains?

Coping strategies to manage labor pains are taught in great detail in childbirth classes. The most common strategies include massage, breathing techniques, and counterpressure. Counterpressure is the application of pressure (by your support person), usually against the sacrum, the back, and the hips to provide pain relief and to help your back feel supported. Be sure to let your support person know where it feels best and how much pressure to use. Another common recommendation is to remain active during labor instead of lying in bed. Some childbirth classes will recommend swaying with a partner, walking around a bit if you're able to stand, or even just switching positions in bed—basically, listen to your body and move in ways that feel best to you. One of the most sought-after strategies is the use of hydrotherapy. Whether in the shower or a birth tub, this is known to help manage the pain of labor tremendously. Typically, you should not enter the water until an active labor pattern has been established because the relaxation from water is so effective that it can slow labor down.

Q. What are the different types of pushing?

There are several different types of pushing that can be used for birth. Without medication, most people will use "instinctive pushing" because the baby pushing against the rectal nerves causes an involuntary urge to push. If you are giving birth for the first time, even without medication, "coached pushing," or help directing your energy to where you need to push and for how long, can be helpful.

For those who have an epidural, most hospitals will have you "labor down," a technique that takes advantage of the uterus naturally pushing the baby further into the pelvis without exerting much physical effort so you can conserve energy for the final stretch of labor. Even if you're at 10 centimeters, hospital staff may wait until the baby is very low until they direct you to push. It is very common practice in a hospital setting to utilize stirrups and coached pushing, which is also sometimes referred to as "purple pushing." This usually entails holding your breath to 10 and pushing three times during a contraction. The birthing person's lips can turn purple from holding their breath too long while pushing. Talk to your care provider and see what they find most effective so you know your options and what you would like to try in labor.

Q. What are the different positions I can push in? What are the advantages/disadvantages of each position?

The positions you can push in are tied to your range of mobility, which is based on whether you're medicated. If you have an epidural, you're limited to pushing on your back or side. In some cases, the anesthesia wears off and you can push on the bed with a squat bar or by leaning over the back of the hospital bed on your hands and knees. In home or birth-center settings, usually anything is game. From semi-reclining in the birth tub, to hands and knees, to side lying, to squatting in a door, there are many variations of what intuitively feels right in order to open up to push your baby out. Pelvic-floor physical therapists are trained to feel what position the pelvic floor is most relaxed in prior to birth, so if you see one prior to giving birth, this knowledge can be helpful. However, I encourage being intuitive in the moment regardless of what the testing showed.

The most important thing to remember is anything that opens the pelvis will be most beneficial. Research shows that squatting while pushing opens the pelvic outlet by an extra 20 to 30 percent, allowing the sacrum and coccyx to move out of the way. If you're in a bed, try to move frequently side to side without putting too much pressure on your back.

Q. What is an episiotomy, and why would I need one?

An episiotomy is a surgical technique where a care provider uses surgical instruments, usually scissors, to make an incision into the perineum (the skin between your vulva and anus) in an attempt to open it up. Since 2006 the American College of Obstetricians and Gynecologists has stated that this procedure should be used sparingly, and as a result it is something we're seeing less and less. If you have an older care provider who is used to performing these routinely, remember you have the right to refuse this procedure. There is a high rate of dissatisfaction with healing and trauma with episiotomies and an increase in pain with intercourse. All in all, it is (or should be!) common knowledge that episiotomies should only be used in emergency situations.

Q. Is there anything I can do to prevent tearing?

Many people will read that doing perineal massage can help reduce tearing, and while this might be true, one of the most important things you can do is use breath awareness during this massage in the prenatal period to help you learn how to relax these muscles. The best way to do this is by utilizing a pelvic-floor physical therapist. They will tell you exactly what tissue is too tight or too loose and how to perform perineal massage. If you don't have access to a pelvic-floor physical therapist, you or your partner can perform this massage using food-grade oil or a carrier oil mixed with your favorite type of mild essential oil, like lavender. With clean hands, gently put one or two fingers into your vagina, taking your fingers down to your perineum, which is the bottom part of the opening of your vagina, by your anus. Once you feel a little bit of pressure, take a deep breath down into this tissue and try to soften it. The purpose of this is aware-ness, not stretching.

Q. What are the different degrees of vaginal tearing, and how are they handled?

There are four degrees of vaginal tearing. The first degree is through the tissue of the perineum. The second is through the tissue and muscle of the perineum. The third is through the tissue, muscle, and to the top of the anus. The fourth is through the anus. First-degree tears may or may not require a few stitches and have a pretty simple recovery. The deeper tears usually require more reconstructive stitch-ing repair and much more intense healing. Witch hazel pads can be very beneficial in the recovery process, and pelvic-floor physical therapy (see page 82) is imperative to help with the healing process.

Q. What is an assisted delivery, and why would I need one?

This is also referred to as an operative vaginal delivery. It means that a device—a vacuum or forceps—is used to help the baby be born quickly through the vagina. A vacuum assist involves attach-ing a plastic suction cup to the top of the baby's head, and a forceps delivery involves placing a pair of forceps carefully on the sides of the baby's head. While you push, the operator pulls on the vacuum device or maneuvers the forceps to provide a little extra help to get the baby out. Some operative vaginal deliveries are performed in cases of emergency where the birth needs to happen quickly—for example, if the baby's heartbeat slows down repeatedly or for a pro-longed period of time. In other cases, operative deliveries are done because the birthgiver is getting exhausted and can't push effectively anymore. One reason that pushing the baby out can take longer than normal is if the baby is not in the ideal position in the birth canal. In these cases, an operative delivery may help turn the baby into the optimal position, which then allows the birth to occur. Operative delivery does have some risks, so it's a judgment call as to when to resort to one of these methods. Keep in mind, though, that an operative vaginal delivery in some situations may have less risk than a cesarean.

Q. *What are the most common medical indications that a cesarean birth is the best option?*

In many cases, it's hard to say for sure that cesarean is *the best* option. What *is* possible is to describe the various reasons why cesareans are recommended. The most common reason for the first cesarean delivery is poor progress in labor (dilating slowly or not at all), but guidelines have changed to allow more time in labor so that now fewer cesareans are performed for this reason. A second common reason for cesarean delivery during labor is concerns about changes in the baby's heart rate. The problem is that providers vary widely in terms of when they recommend a cesarean. Some doctors recommend a cesarean after observing minor abnormalities in the baby's heart rate, while others require more significant abnormalities for longer periods of time before resorting to surgery. There are national efforts to try to standardize these decisions, but despite these efforts, there is still pretty wide variation in how providers manage fetal heart rate abnormalities in labor. Another common reason for cesarean birth is if you have already had a cesarean in a prior pregnancy. Although vaginal birth after cesarean (VBAC) is a reasonable option in most cases, the reality is that for those who have had a cesarean before, currently over 90 percent will have a repeat cesarean in their next pregnancy, either by choice or because they can't find a provider or hospital that will support them in their decision to have a VBAC. There are other situations, like twins or breech presentation, where OB doctors will commonly recommend delivery via cesarean, even though vaginal birth may be a perfectly good or even preferable option.

Q. Will future pregnancies be impacted by a previous cesarean?

The vast majority of the time, subsequent pregnancies after a previous cesarean have no related complications. However, there are some issues that can occur. One of the main decisions you will need to make is whether you would prefer to try for a vaginal birth after cesarean (VBAC) or schedule a repeat cesarean. Both options are safe overall, but both have small risks of potentially serious complications. Recovery from vaginal birth is usually faster and easier, and breastfeeding is also more likely to be successful. If you have a successful VBAC, you have a high chance of having a VBAC again if you have more children. The main risk with VBAC is that the cesarean scar on the uterus can tear open while you're in labor. This happens in less than 1 percent of labors if there is only one prior cesarean, but it can be a very serious complication. Repeat cesarean avoids this risk and also avoids having to labor at all, but a cesarean surgery has risks of its own. In addition to the usual risks of surgery like heavy bleeding, internal organ injuries, serious internal infections, wound complications, blood clots in your leg veins or lungs, and prolonged recovery, breastfeeding and bonding with your baby may be more challenging due to the healing incision on your belly. Beyond these risks, there is a placental condition known as placenta accreta that happens mainly in those who have had one or more prior cesareans. See page 172 for a discussion of this condition.

Q. If I have a cesarean birth, what can I expect?

This will depend on whether you have a planned cesarean or an unplanned one. Many hospitals are now adopting polices to incorporate a "gentle or family-centered" cesarean, so do your research if that is of interest to you (more on page 126).

PLANNED CESAREAN
The night before the cesarean you will stop eating and drinking at midnight. If you're taking medications, you should take them on

schedule with a small sip of water, even on the morning of surgery. If you're taking medications for diabetes, ask for specific instructions from your doctor. You will usually arrive with your support person a couple of hours before the scheduled surgery to get registered, have an IV placed, and meet with the anesthesiologist. Pubic hair is usually trimmed before a cesarean because this has been shown to reduce the chances of surgical infections. At some point prior to surgery a bladder catheter is inserted. If you have any remaining questions, you will have the opportunity to ask them. Once it's time, you will usually enter into the OR with the labor and delivery team while your support person waits just outside. After the spinal or epidural has been placed and is confirmed to be working well, your support person will be brought in to sit with you during the birth. The lower half of your body will go numb and you will not be able to move your legs. This numbness will wear off within about four hours. You will be connected to various monitors like an EKG monitor, blood pressure cuff, and oxygen sensor. After setup is complete and the anesthesia is working well, your belly will be cleaned with a sterilizing soap. A surgical drape (like a blanket) is then placed over you to keep the surgical field sterile. The end of the drape that is near your head is held up on IV poles so that you can't see your belly or the surgery during the operation. A dose of antibiotics is given to reduce the chances of surgical infections. During the cesarean, you may feel uncomfortable lying flat on your back, but this should get better after your baby is born. Sometimes the anesthesia can cause some nausea and vomiting, but the anesthesiologist will be able to address that issue quickly if it happens. You should not feel any sharp cutting, but you may feel the pressure of hands on you, slight body movements, and perhaps some pulling sensations. If you're very nervous or feeling more than you want to be feeling during the cesarean, the anesthesiologist can give you additional medications. The only downside to these IV medications is that you may be drowsy for a couple of hours and may not be awake enough for skin-to-skin baby bonding and breastfeeding right after the cesarean. A cesarean will usually take somewhere between 30 and 60 minutes. The baby is usually born early on in the procedure, and the remainder of the time is spent delivering the placenta, controlling any bleeding, and closing the uterine and skin incisions. After the procedure is done, you will usually be moved to a nearby surgical recovery area for an hour or two of close monitoring before moving to your postpartum room.

UNPLANNED CESAREAN

An unplanned cesarean can happen if you're in labor and trying for a vaginal birth but need a cesarean for some unexpected reason (see page 121 for medical reasons for cesarean). You could also go into labor before your scheduled surgery date, requiring your cesarean to be done sooner. Most unplanned cesareans are performed in a calm, orderly fashion, and all the steps that are outlined previously happen in pretty much the same way. Your support person should be able to sit with you during the surgery. If an epidural is already in place it can most often be used for the cesarean as long as it has been working well. In these cases, the anesthesiologist gives an extra dose of medications through the epidural catheter, and the lower half of the body is numbed for surgery. If the cesarean needs to be done quickly because of a sudden emergency, then the same steps will be followed but very quickly. Also, the support person may not be able to go into the OR with you for the procedure. If you have to be put to sleep with general anesthesia, your support person will definitely have to wait for you outside the OR. After the surgery, if it was done under spinal or epidural anesthesia, hopefully things will be calm, and you will be able to do skin-to-skin baby bonding and start breastfeeding. If the cesarean is done under general anesthesia, you will wake up right away after the surgery is over, but you will likely feel groggy for a few hours. This may cause a delay in skin-to-skin baby bonding and breastfeeding.

Q. What are the benefits versus the risks of a cesarean?

The benefits of a cesarean include knowing when your birth will be (if it is planned) and avoidance of the pain and risks that come with labor and childbirth. It may also be the safest way to deliver your baby in a few specific situations (although vaginal birth is the safest in most cases). There are certain situations where the safety of vaginal birth and cesarean are comparable, making cesarean a reasonable choice. Examples include prior cesarean or a breech-presenting baby (when the baby is positioned bottom-down, or feet first, instead of head-down). Some studies show that cesarean delivery decreases the chances of pelvic-floor disorders like urinary incontinence (involuntary leakage of urine), but this benefit appears to be mainly in the first year after the birth, and the difference fades over time.

There are short-term and long-term risks for you and baby from cesarean. Short-term risks to you are things like hemorrhage, injury to internal organs, surgical infections, formation of blood clots in the legs or lungs, incision complications, and pain. Many people think that a cesarean avoids the pain of childbirth, but studies show that those who deliver by cesarean have more pain overall, both at the time of birth and even months to years later. Babies born by cesarean have a higher chance of breathing difficulties immediately after birth, and occasionally a baby gets cut by the scalpel during delivery.

Long term, the main risks occur during future pregnancies. Subsequent pregnancies are at slightly higher risk for severe complications, either during an attempted vaginal birth or during a repeat cesarean. Future pregnancies are at dramatically higher risk for serious complications if placenta accreta occurs. For the child who is delivered by cesarean, there appear to be some long-term risks, such as increased chances of asthma, allergies, obesity, diabetes, and autoimmune conditions. Another issue is that breastfeeding may be less successful after a cesarean; therefore, the baby may lose out on some of the many health benefits of breastfeeding. In the first year after birth, babies born by cesarean appear to get sick and be hospitalized more often than children born vaginally. Whether the cesarean itself or other factors are causing these complications is not yet known for sure.

Q. What is a gentle or family-centered cesarean?

In a gentle cesarean, the idea is to try to make the birth feel less medical and to preserve as many of the natural processes that happen during vaginal birth as possible. This is a relatively new concept, and not all doctors and hospitals do these things. In a gentle cesarean, more than one support person might be allowed into the operating room with you. In a traditional cesarean, your arms are loosely strapped to the arm boards on the operating table to prevent you from accidentally contaminating the sterile field. In a gentle cesarean, the arm straps are removed so you can hold your baby, or perhaps your arms aren't strapped down at all.

During the birth itself, the drapes may be lowered so that you can actually see your baby being born. Some hospitals have clear drapes that you can see through. A few OB surgeons allow the uterus to push the baby out naturally rather than pulling the baby out in the traditional way. When the baby comes out, cord clamping can be delayed as is often done in a vaginal birth. Studies have shown this to be safe and beneficial for the baby even during a cesarean. Finally, and perhaps most importantly, rather than taking the baby to the nursery, the baby may be left with you and your support team. If you're feeling up for it, skin-to-skin bonding can happen while the surgeon is finishing up the cesarean. Overall, the goal is to minimize separation of you and your baby as much as possible.

Q. What is delayed cord clamping?

This is the practice of not clamping or cutting the umbilical cord until it has stopped pulsating. If the cord is cut before it stops pulsating, the baby will not receive all of its blood volume, potentially putting it into a hypovolemic state of shock. Dr. Alan Green did a fantastic TED Talk on this topic about how something so simple can actually reduce infant mortality—I suggest looking it up if you're interested.

Q. What are the benefits of consuming my placenta, and how do I do so?

There is much debate about consuming the placenta after birth. While it's true that many mammals do so, there is no proven benefit to humans, though the placenta is rich in iron, nutrients, and hormones. Many have anecdotally reported a significant difference in mood, milk supply, and energy levels when comparing postpartum periods with and without placenta encapsulation, a process by which the placenta is steamed, dehydrated, ground to powder, and placed into capsules. Your midwife, doula, or doctor may be able to provide a reference for someone who can help you with this service. You want to make sure that your encapsulator takes proper safety precautions of not mixing your placenta with another person's. A good placenta encapsulator will also ask for your prenatal labs to make sure there isn't a reason to not encapsulate. For example, if you are positive for group B strep or there is any concern with infection during the labor or birth, unfortunately your placenta is not a good candidate for encapsulation.

Q. Why might my baby be taken to the NICU?

NICU stands for "neonatal intensive care unit." It is a unit for newborn infants needing specialized care for any reason. The most common reason that babies go to the NICU is for prematurity (birth at less than 37 weeks' gestation). If a baby is born at 34 weeks or fewer, it is almost guaranteed that the baby will be admitted to the NICU, even if the baby looks perfectly strong and healthy at birth. Between 35 and 37 weeks, many babies will be developed enough that they don't need the NICU, although a certain percentage will still need to be admitted. Once you have reached term (37 weeks), the chance that your baby will be in the NICU is much lower. However, even for a term birth, if the baby appears to have difficulty breathing, the baby might go to the NICU for observation or oxygen therapy. If there has been a high fever in labor, the baby might go to the NICU for blood tests (to look for infection) and possibly even antibiotics. If it was a difficult birth, the baby might go to the NICU for observation.

After birth, a baby's bilirubin (a substance released from broken-down red blood cells) may be elevated. This is very common in preemies but can even happen after a full-term birth. If the bilirubin rises to a moderately high level, admission to the NICU may be required for treatment. Sometimes it is known in advance that the baby will be admitted to the NICU after birth. This can happen when the baby is known to have a birth defect that is expected to require treatment right after the birth.

Q. What can I expect as a parent of a baby in the NICU?

If your baby is admitted to the NICU, you will be given specific information about what medical problems your baby is dealing with and what the treatment plan is. When situations are medically complex like this, in addition to the stress and anxiety over the health of the baby, many parents experience a feeling of helplessness. One question all parents have is how long their baby will need to stay in the NICU. If the baby is admitted for prematurity, one rule of thumb is to expect the baby to stay until the baby reaches 36 to 38 weeks. For example, if the birth happens at 30 weeks, expect your baby to stay in the NICU for six to eight weeks. Some babies may be ready for discharge earlier, and some may need more time. Another common question is how often you will be able to visit your baby. Most NICUs allow visits at any time of the day or night. There may be some time slots where families are asked to step out for perhaps an hour or so to allow the medical team to do their rounds. If your baby is admitted to the NICU, you can ask for the exact visiting hours. Keep in mind that babies in the NICU are vulnerable to serious infections, so they try to limit the number of visitors who come into the unit. Don't expect that all of your family and friends will be able to come and see your baby in the NICU.

In terms of the actual medical care, what happens in the NICU depends on what is going on with your baby. Lots of tests are ordered in the NICU, including blood tests, urine tests, x-rays, ultrasounds, and sometimes even CT scans or MRIs. Some babies in the NICU will need surgery for varying reasons. Because these babies are so tiny, it can sometimes look like they are completely covered in wires and lines. Even just the sight of this can be extremely emotionally distressing for parents. In this scenario, you may not be able to pick your baby up until later, but you will always be able to touch your baby. The role of the parent in the NICU is extremely important! Your baby needs to hear your voice and feel your touch (even just holding their little hand or foot if they can't be picked up yet). If your baby can't breastfeed yet, you can still pump and give expressed breast milk. Studies have shown that these interactions with the parents improve outcomes for these delicate little babies, so have faith that you're making a difference.

"The postpartum period is as primal as giving birth. It's all about survival and adjusting to this huge life change. And it has two saving graces: blissed out newborn snuggles and the fact that it's temporary."

—Stephanie Coffield

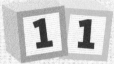

Postpartum Care

*Lindsey Meehleis, LM, CPM
and Courtney Butts, LMSW*

Recovering from childbirth is unlike anything else—your hormones are surging, your body is healing, and on top of all of that, you have a tiny human to take care of! In this chapter you'll find the answers to questions regarding immediate postpartum recovery for you (both mental and physical) and care for your newborn as well as longer-term adjusting to life as a new parent. Sometimes additional concerns arise postpartum; if you're concerned about your health or your baby's, always call your provider right away.

Q. What can I expect right after my baby is born?

This will be different based on the birth you had, your care provider, and your insurance policy. You can typically expect the following:

HOSPITAL

The type of hospital you gave birth in will dictate what follows immediately after the birth. If the baby is pink and vigorous, they can be placed directly on your chest for skin-to-skin bonding. The nurses can do all assessments there, which include the one- and five-minute Apgar scores. Typically, hospital rooms are pretty cold, so be sure when baby is skin to skin to keep blankets over the baby. If the baby is cold, they will bring the baby to the warmer instead of your chest. During this time, also known as the "Golden Hour," they should leave your baby on your chest to get the first breastfeeding established and hold off for that hour on any newborn procedures, like weighing, measuring, and bathing the baby; giving the vitamin K shot; and applying antibiotic eye drops or ointment. All of these newborn procedures are typically mandated by the state, but every hospital should have refusal forms if you choose not to do them. Do your research to see what works best for your family; EvidenceBasedBirth.com is a good resource.

During this time, if you had a perineal tear, the doctor or midwife will suture and repair it. They will watch your bleeding and perform fundal massage, which is where they will rub your uterus to ensure that it is staying firm. In most hospitals, families are moved from the labor and delivery unit to the postpartum unit within a few hours following the birth. Before the move to the postpartum unit, they like to see epidural anesthesia worn off so you can get to the restroom on your own, and they may want you to urinate before changing rooms. The nurse may provide you with a cold pack, witch hazel pads, and mesh underwear for postpartum healing and recovery assistance.

BIRTH CENTER

Most birth centers should be "baby friendly" (see BabyFriendlyUSA. org), but be sure to ask what their afterbirth protocols are, just to be sure. They all typically conform to the same procedures as a hospital but in a different setting. Talk to your midwives regarding what is mandated in your state or country to learn more about what procedures you would or wouldn't like for your baby.

HOME BIRTH

Home births are usually less rushed in terms of getting through post-delivery checklists, but because most newborn procedures are mandated by the state, they will most likely need to be performed at some point. Be sure to check with your midwife or midwives well before the birth to see what you can expect for the postpartum period.

Q. What is the "Golden Hour," and why is it important?

As previously mentioned, the Golden Hour is a period of time for you and your baby to remain together. This means no interruptions unless they're medically indicated. Your baby should be skin to skin with you instead of bundled in blankets or hats, using your body heat to regulate their own, with only a blanket over you and the baby. Plus, you can lift the blankets and start to explore their body, counting fingers and toes. The lights should be low so baby can start to open their eyes, voices in the room should be kept soft, and the first nursing session should be encouraged, either by directly placing baby to the breast or by allowing the baby to "crawl" toward the nipple. Breast crawling is when the baby starts to move its feet, bob its head, and motion toward the nipple. In unmedicated births, it's very possible for babies to find and latch on without any assistance. The Golden Hour also includes delaying any newborn procedures. If the Golden Hour isn't available for circumstances out of your control (cesarean, NICU observation, etc.), it can still be duplicated when you come together for the first time; there will be time to bond. If you're unavailable, your partner can also do skin to skin with the baby during this time.

Q. What newborn tests/screenings will be offered? Are the same tests offered for an out-of-hospital birth?

Typically, you can expect that a newborn metabolic screening test will be performed 48 to 72 hours following the birth. This a nationally mandated test, but there is no national standard—each state has certain criteria it tests for, though you can likely sign a form to decline some portions of the screening. Most hospitals offer a newborn hearing test to detect any hearing problems; most hospitals do this test in the room with you. There is also a rise in screening for congenital heart defects. A pulse oximeter machine is connected to your baby's hand and foot to monitor oxygenation. Remember, none of these are mandatory, so do your research. Every state's screening is different, so check with your care provider to be sure of what is absolutely necessary.

Q. How long does recovery from a vaginal birth take, and what can I expect?

Everyone recovers differently, so we can't put a time frame on this. Listen to your body! If you're doing too much, your body will tell you with an increase in bleeding. The less you do, the faster you heal! You can bleed up to six weeks following the birth (sometimes a little longer), which means you still have an internal wound that is healing, so give yourself some grace. The newborn period passes in the blink of an eye, and the more you rest and spend time getting to know your baby, the smoother and faster your recovery will be.

Q. What do I need to know about that first pee after delivery?

Many hospitals, birth centers, and midwives like to have you pee with assistance after the birth. The baby is finally out of your uterus, and all of your organs have to settle into place, which can leave you feeling out of breath and strange. If you've had an epidural, you're likely feeling sensation in your lower body again but may still be unsteady. It's good to take this slowly; sit on the edge of the bed and gradually get up to go to the bathroom. If you feel faint or light-headed, be sure to tell your care provider and return to bed. There is no shame in peeing in a bedpan. If you have perineal tearing, there might be a slight burning sensation while peeing, so use the peri bottle (a special bottle to help rinse your perineum and aid healing) with either plain water or the herbal infusion they give you to dilute the urine and help ease the burn.

Q. What is a postpartum care kit, and why do I need one?

Good things to put in a postpartum care kit include:

» Maternity or thick menstrual pads.
» Premade witch hazel pads or witch hazel–soaked cotton rounds, which you can freeze to aid in reducing swelling and healing your perineum.
» Mesh underwear, which is often provided by the hospital or your midwife in their birth kit.
» A peri bottle, with herbs to make a vaginal rinse to use when you go to the bathroom.
» A sitz bath (a large bowl that fits on the toilet with a small hose attached to it) that you can sit in or use to rinse yourself with healing herbs and warm water to heal your perineum.

You can buy all of the supplies separately, or you can get them as in a pre-assembled kit online.

Q. What pain medications are safe to take while breastfeeding?

Anything that is prescribed by your doctor or midwife is safe, as they know what medications are contraindicated for breastfeeding. Each provider has a different combination of meds they prescribe; if you're worried, ask for clarification. If you have had a cesarean birth, you will most likely be given stronger medication to help with the pain of recovering from an abdominal surgery. This medication is to be taken on a short-term basis before switching over to ibuprofen. Ibuprofen is the most commonly used pain medication following birth and is safe for breastfeeding.

Q. I had a cesarean birth. What can I expect during my recovery?

Your birth experience prior to surgery will indicate what to expect for recovery. If you were in labor for 48 hours, pushed for three hours, and then had a cesarean, your recovery will be much harder than someone who slept all night and went in for a scheduled cesarean birth. But what you can expect is recovery from major abdominal surgery. You will have to recover from the medication, the incision, and the soreness. They will want you up and walking typically within 24 hours following the birth. This first walk can be painful, so prepare yourself mentally for standing the first time. The recovery is a bit longer for cesarean birth as well. Physical recovery from a vaginal birth is typically about six weeks. Recovery from a C-section may be closer to eight weeks. Keep in mind this is just physical recovery; there are many aspects to healing from a cesarean, especially if it was unplanned. Emotional healing is important, too, and can take much longer. Please seek additional help from a therapist who specializes in maternal mental health or a postpartum support group if you find yourself having trouble processing your feelings about your birth experience.

Q. What is considered normal with postpartum bleeding?

For a vaginal birth you may bleed for up to six weeks; for a cesarean birth, up to eight weeks. The more active you are the more you will bleed, so rest. Take it easy. If you bleed past this point or the blood goes from brown back to bright red or is getting heavier, contact your care provider.

Q. When will I see my doctor or midwife for a postpartum checkup?

Typically, with a vaginal birth a doctor will see you when they discharge you from the hospital and then again at six weeks to discuss birth control options. With a cesarean, you'll see the doctor when you're discharged, at two weeks to check the incision, and then again at six weeks. For midwifery clients, it is common to be seen at 24 to 48 hours, one week, two weeks, and six weeks. There are typically more appointments added if there are breastfeeding issues or if postpartum depression comes up. Follow up with your doctor or midwife to see what their protocol is.

Q. What are signs that I should seek medical help postpartum?

The most important thing is to trust yourself. You know your body better than anyone, so if you have concerns, contact your care provider. Things to look out for include any fever over 100, abnormal/foul-smelling discharge, excessive bleeding, and pain in the uterus outside of the normal uterine cramping. Another thing to pay attention to is your mental health. If you feel that your emotions are more than "baby blues" and you're struggling to take care of yourself or your baby or if you have thoughts about harming yourself or your baby, contact your provider immediately. (More on postpartum mood disorders on pages 139-141.)

Q. How will I know if I need pelvic-floor therapy? How do I find a therapist, and what can I expect at my appointment?

Pelvic-floor physical therapy before and after birth can be very helpful. If you are having any pain in your pelvic floor, incontinence with urination, or pain with intercourse, it is imperative that you seek help to strengthen your pelvic floor. During a typical pelvic-floor appointment, your provider will talk you through what they are going to do, but this is an assessment of the pelvic-floor muscles, so it usually includes a pelvic exam, which can make some people uncomfortable. Be sure to talk to your provider and see if there is anything that can be done to make your exam more comfortable. To find a pelvic-floor therapist, ask your pregnancy care provider or a friend who has recently given birth for a recommendation.

Q. When can I resume exercise after my baby is born?

You can typically resume exercise when uterine bleeding has ceased and you feel healed. Remember, for someone who has had a vaginal birth, this can last up to six weeks, and someone who has had a cesarean will take eight weeks. Check with your care provider to make sure you're cleared, and start slowly. If you start bleeding again, it's too soon. Listen to your body and have fun. You should not feel pressured to "bounce back" after giving birth, so start with an exercise routine that's enjoyable and feels good, like daily walks with your baby.

Q. When is it safe to have sex again postpartum, and what can I expect?

Much like exercise, the general rule is when you have physically recovered and bleeding has stopped. Most care providers recommend waiting six weeks. It is also important to be emotionally ready. Birth can be traumatic, and if you aren't ready, that's okay. Keep in mind that if you're nursing, you have a baby attached to your nipples 10 to 14 times a day, so you might be "touched out." Nursing can also reduce the level of vaginal lubrication that you have, so if you wish to have penetrative sex, you may want to use lubrication for a more pleasant experience. If you're not ready for that, you can find new ways to be intimate with your partner. The important thing is to focus on clear communication with your partner, be open with your feelings—and know that they are normal.

Q. If I'm breastfeeding, do I still need to use birth control?

Not having a period is one of the most effective forms of birth control in the world, but there's a catch: You will ovulate before you know your period has come back. This means that you have the potential to be fertile before you even know your period has returned. Some parents remain in amenorrhea (have no period) for as long as they nurse, and others get their cycle back right away. Talk to your care provider about safe forms of non-hormonal birth control, and consider reading the book *Taking Charge of Your Fertility* by Toni Weschler.

Q. I'm super-emotional and weepy. Is this normal?

Yes! You're not alone! Approximately 80 percent of all birthing people experience the "baby blues" in the first few days after giving birth. Baby blues are due to drastic hormonal shifts and are often described as feelings of worry and fatigue that come from the pressure of providing for a newborn.

After childbirth, your hormone levels decrease drastically; coupled with lack of sleep, these changes can contribute to symptoms such as irritability, mood swings, and crying spells. While these feelings are normal, they can often be overwhelming.

Symptoms typically resolve once hormones return to pre-pregnancy levels, typically around two to three weeks after your baby is born. While mild mood changes are common, symptoms can sometimes become severe enough to require treatment. If feelings of depression or anxiety persist for a few weeks or interfere with daily activities, it's time to ask for help.

Q. What are the warning signs for postpartum mood disorders?

Are you feeling sad or depressed? How about anxious or irritable? Some new parents have difficulty bonding with their baby or feel out of control. These are all possible warning signs for postpartum mood disorders. While symptoms vary, if you're feeling "not like yourself" during the postpartum period, it's important to check in with your care provider or a licensed mental health specialist.

POSTPARTUM DEPRESSION (PPD)

Approximately 15 to 20 percent of birthing people experience depression during the postpartum period. This number is even higher for families of color and can double for teen parents. Postpartum depression symptoms may include feelings of anger, intense sadness, worthlessness, changes in eating or sleeping habits, or lack of interest in the baby. These feelings get in the way of daily life and can occur up to one year after your baby arrives.

POSTPARTUM ANXIETY (PPA)

Postpartum anxiety impacts approximately 10 percent of all birthing people. Symptoms include constant worry and racing thoughts, including feeling as if something bad is going to happen. Postpartum anxiety can also include:

» Panic attacks, or a sudden rush of fear that includes sweating, a racing heart, shortness of breath, chest pain, and/or fear of losing control.
» Obsessions, or unwanted and intrusive thoughts or impulses that cause distress.
» Compulsive rituals or repetitive behaviors designed to reduce stress, like washing, checking, and seeking reassurance, which are usually a response to an obsession.
» Persistent concern and worry about the future, including thoughts about the "worst case scenario."

POST-TRAUMATIC STRESS DISORDER (PTSD)

Post-traumatic stress disorder (PTSD), often caused by experiencing or witnessing a traumatic event, may result in reexperiencing the trauma, including flashbacks. Impacting about 9 percent of birthing people following childbirth, symptoms may include:

» Recurrent and intrusive thoughts or images or nightmares of the traumatic event, which can be the childbirth itself.
» Avoidance of thoughts, feelings, people, and places related to the trauma.
» Persistent arousal, including difficulty concentrating, sleep disturbances, hypervigilance, and irritability.

POSTPARTUM PSYCHOSIS

A new parent experiencing postpartum psychosis may see or hear voices that others cannot, may believe things that are not true, or may have a high level of distrust. There is a serious risk of the parent hurting themselves or their baby. This is a severe mental health condition and requires immediate medical attention.

Q. Where can I go for help if I suspect I might have postpartum mood disorder?

First, know that you're not to blame. You're also not alone. If you suspect you may have a postpartum mood disorder, please check in with a care provider you trust. Your OBGYN, midwife, primary care physician, or pediatrician or a licensed mental health professional can help with diagnosis and treatment options. Postpartum Support International has several support options, including a telephone helpline (1-800-944-4773) and text line (503-894-9453), or you can visit Postpartum.net to find local support groups in your area. If you're in crisis or in an emergency, please call your local emergency number or the National Suicide Prevention Hotline at 1-800-273-8255.

You can also use an assessment tool called the Edinburgh Postnatal Depression Scale (fresno.ucsf.edu/pediatrics/downloads/edinburghscale.pdf). This is a 10-question survey used to assess for postpartum depression. If you're worried about how you're feeling, it may be helpful to complete this assessment and take the results to a trusted doctor or licensed mental health professional to discuss treatment options.

Q. How will my care provider diagnose me with a postpartum mood disorder?

Your provider may begin by asking questions about your symptoms, home life, and mental health history. Be open and honest about your feelings and experiences. There are several screening tools your care provider may use to assess for mood disorders. Your provider may also use the Diagnostic and Statistical Manual of Mental Disorders to review the diagnostic criteria for mood and anxiety disorders.

If your provider determines that you have a postpartum mood disorder, you will work together to find the best treatment options to relieve your symptoms.

Q. What are my treatment options for postpartum mood disorders?

Help is available to treat postpartum mood and anxiety disorders. It's important to seek professional help in addition to support from family and friends.

» Psychotherapy, also known as talk therapy, is an effective treatment option for individuals or couples.
» Group therapy can help new parents feel less isolated through social interactions. It can also provide a safe and accepting space for parents to process their birth experience and parenthood without shame or judgment.
» Intensive outpatient and partial hospitalization programs.
» Medications are also an option. If you're nursing, the idea of medication can be frightening, but there are many medications that are safe for breastfeeding parents. Work closely with your care provider to decide if medication is the best course of treatment for you.

Q. Are there medications I can take for PPD/PPA that are safe while breastfeeding?

Yes. Although medications can pose potential risks, in some cases, they are an important and effective treatment option while nursing. It is important to talk to your care provider in order to make an informed decision about what's best for you and your baby. You can visit InfantRisk.com for more information about medication safety during pregnancy and while breastfeeding.

Q. What online and phone resources are available for postpartum mental health support?

POSTPARTUM SUPPORT INTERNATIONAL (PSI)
» 1-800-944-4773
» postpartum.net
» Send a text to 503-894-9453 for the PSI Helpline

NATIONAL CRISIS TEXT LINE
» Text HOME to 741741

NATIONAL SUICIDE PREVENTION HOTLINE
» 1-800-273-8255
» suicidepreventionlifeline.org

Q. Are certain people more at risk than others of developing a postpartum mood disorder?

Risk for postpartum mood and anxiety disorders increases significantly for new parents who have had a personal or family history of depression or anxiety, ambivalence about being a parent, or inadequate support from family and friends. Other risk factors include:

» Recent stress
» Absent or unsupportive partner
» Past trauma history

» Previous loss
» Absence of social support
» Complications during pregnancy, delivery, or both
» Premature delivery and NICU families
» Unwanted pregnancy
» Infertility issues
» Financial problems
» Being LGBTQ+

Q. My birth was traumatic. How do I find help processing what happened?

The birth of a child can be a magical experience, but it can also be one of the most frightening. For some, the experience of labor and delivery can be traumatic and even triggering of past trauma, even when labor goes according to plan. During labor, you can feel out of control, fearful for your baby's safety, overwhelmed with the pain of labor, unprepared, unsupported by friends or family, or triggered by a previous traumatic delivery.

It is common to experience many feelings and emotions after a stressful event like childbirth. However, if you continue to have intrusive flashbacks or nightmares about the birth, feel emotionally detached from the baby, or avoid talking about childbirth, then you may be experiencing a post-traumatic stress response. Please reach out to a mental health professional for further support in processing your feelings.

Seeking help from a mental health professional can seem over-whelming. The goal of treatment is to improve your symptoms and help develop healthy coping skills. There are several evidence-based modalities a trained mental health professional can use to help you process your trauma/PTSD. They will evaluate your situation and choose the method that's right for you.

Q. How can I find a therapist who specializes in perinatal mental health?

Postpartum Support International (PSI, postpartum.net) has a list of providers who specialize in perinatal mental health. Your health care provider may also have a list of perinatal mental health providers in your area.

Q. What are some easy self-care things I can focus on daily?

It may seem strange to prioritize self-care while there's a newborn to care for, but taking care of yourself is one of the most important things you can do as a new parent. It can help relieve any stress you might be feeling, reenergize you, and help you be present for your baby. Some things you can do are:

» Take alone time for yourself or do something that's just for you.
» Go out with friends, even for a short period of time.
» Talk about the stress you're experiencing.
» Get rest whenever you can.
» Allow your partner, family, and friends to help.
» Get up and move around—exercise can boost your energy levels and reduce stress.
» Stay hydrated and consume nutritious foods.

Q. How can I support my partner or a friend who has a postpartum mood disorder?

Emotional difficulties during pregnancy and after the delivery of the baby are common. For most birthing people, symptoms of "baby blues" will resolve without treatment. However, when a new parent develops a postpartum mood disorder, it isn't a problem a person can decide to control. Telling someone it's "not that bad" or to "cheer up" may be well intentioned, but it can be harmful. While it may be difficult to see the new parent going through this experience, your desire to "fix" things may not be helpful. Listen to how they are feeling, and remind them that you care and that you're there for support.

You can also offer practical help. This can look different depending on your situation but can include everything from offering to hold the baby or feeding and changing the baby to preparing a meal, cleaning the house, or doing the laundry and dishes. Postpartum mood disorders also require support and often treatment. Due to the stigma, new parents are often reluctant to seek help; as a member of the support team, educate yourself on the signs and symptoms as well the resources in your area.

Q. *I'm having a difficult time with breastfeeding, and it's affecting my mental health. What should I do?*

Your breastfeeding relationship with your baby should be mutual—it isn't just about the baby. If you're not benefiting from the relationship, you have every right to make changes, especially if it's impacting your mental health. If you would like to continue your breastfeeding relationship, contact a professional in your area for further support. You can visit La Leche League at llli.org for additional information and support in your area.

There is often a lot of pressure placed on the nursing parent to exclusively breastfeed—do not ever feel bad or guilty about not wanting to or not being able to breastfeed your baby. What is most important is the baby is receiving adequate nutrition—from a breast or a bottle. Every parent's situation is unique; lifestyle, work schedule, or medication use can all have an impact on a parent's choice to breastfeed their child.

"I found that all the Googling in the world couldn't prepare me for taking care of my brand new human. Sure, it helped, but what I figured out quickly was that each baby is different and wants and needs different things. Learn your baby's cues and respond to them."

—Ellen Powell

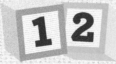

Feeding and Caring for Your Newborn

Lindsey Meehleis, LM, CPM
and Bryn Huntpalmer

Your baby is here—and you're responsible for their every need! If that sentence sounds daunting, well, that's because it can feel daunting to be a new parent, especially when you're sleep-deprived. In this chapter, I and our midwife, Lindsey, will cover newborn basics, including things to be aware of immediately after birth, caring for your baby, and what to expect when it comes to their sleeping, eating, and pooping (because that's about all they do!). You'll also find key advice for feeding your newborn.

Q. How do I care for my baby's umbilical cord stump, and when will it fall off?

Each care practitioner might tell you different things, but the general rule of thumb with umbilical cord care is to keep it dry. As gross as it sounds, this is a piece of flesh that is dying and will eventually fall off. If the cord gets goopy or smelly, you can take a cotton swab and clean the base with rubbing alcohol or hydrogen peroxide. The process of it falling off can take anywhere from two days to two weeks. If the skin becomes inflamed and red around the base of the cord, let your care provider know.

Q. Is this normal? What is going on with my baby's poop?

Immediately following the birth of your baby, you can expect to see a black, tarry poop called meconium. Your baby is born with this poop already in their intestinal tract and passes this at birth or soon after. There should be at least one meconium poop in the first 24-hour period. As this poop transitions from the black tarry substance, you will see it range from brown to green to yellow. If you're breastfeeding, once your milk is fully in, you will start to notice this poop turn into a mustard yellow with some seed-like specks in it. The poop should remain that color until solid foods or formula is introduced. If you see green poop consistently, it could be an imbalance of your hindmilk and foremilk. You can seek lactation help on how to remedy this with ease. If you are formula feeding, your baby's poop will be more of a pasty consistency that is brown—and it can change from a more yellow-based brown to a more green-based brown.

Q. How often should my baby pee and poop?

For the first few days, the general rule of thumb is that baby should produce the same number of wet and poopy diapers as the days since birth, so one wet and one poopy diaper in the first 24 hours, two wet and two poopy diapers in the second 24 hours, and so on. Typically, by day four, your milk has fully transitioned from colostrum and the size of baby's stomach has grown, and from here on out, it's normal to see five to six wet diapers per day and three to four poopy diapers per day (and sometimes many more). Some babies also poop less, and that is still within normal limits. If you have any concerns, contact your pediatrician or a lactation specialist if you are breastfeeding. Formula-fed babies tend to poop less frequently than breast milk–fed babies because it is a heavier protein and moves through the intestines more slowly. At the beginning, they poop up to three to four times daily, but it isn't uncommon after the first few weeks to have them go longer between poops, sometimes up to seven days. As long as your baby's poop isn't formed like hard little pellets, you likely don't have to worry about constipation—but contact your care provider if you are concerned or if your baby seems uncomfortable.

Q. What do I need to know about caring for and cleaning my baby's penis?

This will differ depending on whether your baby is circumcised or intact.

CIRCUMCISION CARE

Typically, the head (glans) of the circumcised penis is covered with gauze and petroleum jelly until the incision has healed to protect it from exposure to feces. Be sure to ask the care provider who performed the circumcision their recommendations on the proper care and cleaning for your child's circumcised penis.

INTACT FORESKIN CARE

For the care of an intact penis, there isn't much to do. The head of the penis (glans) is meant to be an internal organ, and the foreskin protects it. At this stage of development, there is a membrane between the foreskin and the glans that keeps the foreskin from retracting; this is normal. DO NOT retract the foreskin or let any care provider do so; the foreskin will naturally start to retract on its own between the ages of three and six years. Simply wipe away any debris that might be on the penis.

Q. What do I need to know about caring for my baby's vulva and vagina?

One of the most shocking things to parents is that it is normal for a newborn's vulva to produce a white, thick discharge and even small blood-tinged discharge in the first few days. The baby received a hormonal boost at the end of the pregnancy, and these hormones can produce what is colloquially known as "first menstruation." Rest assured—this is totally normal and usually goes away in about a day or two. As for cleaning, there is no need to enter the vagina. Just take a wet cloth or wipe and gently remove any debris on the vulva. It's also a good idea to begin the practice of wiping from front to back, which you'll want to eventually teach your child to do during potty training, too.

Q. What are some quick tips for newborn hygiene that I need to know?

NEWBORN BATHS

Giving newborns baths is a little like bathing a wiggling, wet fish—it's hard! Be sure to take your time, have everything you need right next to you, and be prepared for possible tears, maybe from both of you. Laying a towel down in the tub or sink is also helpful in minimizing slipperiness. My (Lindsey's) favorite time with my own new babies was taking baths together. You can even add herbs to the bath— which can help with your healing, if you had a vaginal birth, and baby's umbilical cord healing as well.

TRIMMING BABY'S NAILS

Again, this is not an easy task. With newborns the easiest way to trim their nails is to file them down. Their nails are so thin that sometimes even tearing them to the side or biting them off is easier than trying to cut them. A good time to try this is while they are eating or sleeping.

CLEARING THE NASAL PASSAGES

Newborns typically keep their nasal passages clear on their own, but if you're noticing extra snot, the best product on the market to keep them clear is the NoseFrida. (Don't let the description gross you out!) If your baby has boogers, you won't be the first parent to pick your baby's nose. Another good option is to use a cool-mist humidifier in the room where the baby sleeps.

Q. What are the symptoms of and treatment for newborn jaundice?

The main signs and symptoms of newborn jaundice are yellowing of the eyes and skin. Jaundice typically is first visible in the whites of the eyes and then moves to the face, into the trunk of the body, and next into the extremities. Your pediatrician or your care provider will assess your newborn, and if the jaundice is severe enough, your baby might be hospitalized under UV lights for treatment. Frequent nursing and indirect sunlight for 15-minute increments, three times a day, can also help move the bilirubin out of your baby's system, lessening the need for medical treatment.

Q. What do I need to know about newborn thrush?

Receiving IV antibiotics in labor can greatly increase the chances of newborn thrush. Thrush is basically a yeast infection of the mouth, nipples, and sometimes diaper area. If you have thrush, you will usually experience burning, red nipples that stay this way between feeds. You might also notice a while, milky substance that coats the baby's mouth but doesn't wipe away. Thrush is not fun to have and can be tricky to treat. Since yeast thrives off sugar, first things first is cutting sugar from your diet. There are prescription and over-the-counter anti-fungal medications that can be used to treat thrush. If you think either you or your baby is experiencing thrush, seek assistance from a lactation specialist.

Q. Do newborns have a typical schedule I should follow?

Not really. A better word than schedule is rhythm. You will learn your baby's rhythm, and it will ebb and flow as the days change. Typically, you will be nursing every one to three hours over a 24-hour period. You're learning each other, so set your expectations low and give yourself a lot of grace. We recommend the Taking Cara Babies newborn class (TakingCaraBabies.com) if you are someone who wants some semblance of a schedule.

Q. How many hours of sleep should my baby get?

Babies sleep a lot in the newborn phase, but every baby is different, so don't set a certain expectation. The average newborn sleeps eight to nine hours a day and eight hours at night, which leaves just a few awake hours to feed, poop, and maybe eye gaze and coo with parents. Take advantage of naps, even though it sounds like a lot; if you aren't sleeping while they are, the broken sleep at night might catch up with you.

Q. My baby hiccups a lot. Do I need to treat their hiccups?

Hiccups are normal. Chances are if your baby hiccupped a lot in utero, they will hiccup a lot on the outside, too. There is no need to treat the hiccups, but if your baby is fussy and you're breastfeeding, you might consider eliminating top allergens (dairy, gluten, eggs) from your diet to see if what you're passing through your milk might be upsetting their tummy.

Q. My baby's skin is breaking out. What should I do?

Nothing. Baby acne is very common in the first two to four weeks of life, although some babies can get it later than four weeks. There's no firm understanding of what causes baby acne, though some believe it to be a result of your hormones from pregnancy. It will go away on its own without any treatment.

Q. What is cradle cap, and how do I treat it?

Cradle cap is a dandruff-like, crusty scale that sometimes happens on the top of your baby's head. It is usually caused by an overactive oil-producing gland. It is reported that up to 70 percent of newborns have experienced this by the age of three months. While you don't have to do anything to treat cradle cap, you can mix a carrier oil with a gentle anti-fungal essential oil like lavender or geranium and softly massage it into your baby's scalp.

Q. How can I tell if my newborn is hungry?

If you watch your newborn, you will learn their hunger cues. Crying is the last sign of hunger, so look for signs of your baby starting to root (make sucking motions when their lips or cheeks are touched). They will bring their hands to their mouth, bob their head up and down, and step their feet. If you respond when you start noticing these signs, you will likely avoid latching or trying to bottle feed a frantic baby, which makes it so much easier.

Q. How often do newborns eat?

FORMULA-FED BABIES

Formula is made from a heavier protein than breast milk, so it takes longer to digest, which makes babies typically eat closer to every three hours. But always listen to your baby; if they are showing hunger cues, feed them.

BREASTFED BABIES

Breastfed babies should be fed on demand, which is typically every two to three hours, or eight to 12 times in a 24-hour period. There are some babies who are fast-food feeders and can empty the breast within five minutes and others who take their time, taking up to 45 minutes to eat. As long as your needs are met and you aren't experiencing nipple pain, it's fine to let them nurse for these longer stretches. If you need a break, though, most babies get the majority of their feeds in about 10 minutes on each side. You can consult a lactation professional for advice. Breastfed babies also cluster feed, which means they stock up on calories before they go into a longer period of sleep. You might notice them feeding every hour or so for a few hours. It's nice to have this cluster feed before bedtime so you can get a longer stretch of sleep at night. Start offering the breast frequently about three hours before you go to bed to see if you can get this cluster feed to occur around that time.

Q. If I'm formula feeding, how do I know which formula to get?

In the United States, infant formula is regulated by the FDA, and all formulas are basically the same. The main thing to consider is whether your formula is dairy-based, soy-based, or protein hydrolysate (also called hypoallergenic). You may also want to consider organic or non-GMO options if that's important to you. Ready-to-feed liquid formulas are sterile and generally considered safer for newborns than the powdered form. If you're using powdered formula, be sure you're following safe preparation guidelines and using filtered water. The CDC has guidelines on preparing infant formula at CDC.gov. If your baby is fussy with a certain type of formula, talk to your pediatrician to see what new formulas you might want to try.

Q. What should I know about bottle feeding?

IF EXCLUSIVELY BOTTLE FEEDING

Offer a bottle at a time when your baby is calm or showing the very first signs of hunger (rooting, squirming, smacking their lips). If you wait until they are upset and hungry, it can be harder to feed them a bottle, and they may also swallow more air. Start with a small amount of breast milk or formula and then give more if they are still showing signs of hunger. Offer the bottle at an angle so they have to actively suck to get milk rather than it just dripping in if the bottle were straight up and down. Pause to burp your baby about halfway through by propping them up on your lap with your hand supporting their head or laying them on your shoulder with your hand on their back and head.

Never force a baby to finish a bottle; if they are constantly popping off the bottle or turning their head away, stop the feeding and try again later. Never prop a bottle up for your baby or leave them unattended with a bottle. Another trick is to treat bottle feeding like breastfeeding, so when bottle feeding, try to switch sides on which your baby lies and bring them in close to you. This will help your baby use both sides of their neck muscles and develop their eyes from looking at you from different angles. You will want to be sure to sterilize your bottles, which you can do by boiling them. More info on formula, safe handling of breast milk, and cleaning infant feeding items is available at CDC.gov. We have a free video at TheBirthHour.com/bottle that shows how and when to introduce a bottle.

IF COMBINING WITH BREASTFEEDING

If your goal is to alternate between breastfeeding and bottle feeding, it's a good idea for your bottle feeding to mimic breastfeeding as much as possible so baby doesn't develop a preference for the bottle over the breast. Be sure to use a slow-flow nipple (stage 1 or even preemie) so baby can't drain the bottle too quickly. You can also practice paced bottle feeding, where you have the baby take little breaks throughout the feed—we have a free video at TheBirthHour.com/bottle that shows how to do this.

Q. What is colostrum, and when will my regular milk come in?

Colostrum is the milk that pregnant people make throughout their pregnancies and for the first few days of baby's life. It's sometimes referred to as "liquid gold" because it's very yellow/gold in physical appearance and because it's dense in nutrients and antibodies, making it the perfect food for the first few days of life. Your baby's stomach is the size of a shooter marble until about day three or day four, and this dense milk provides the baby exactly what they need. Up to two-thirds of the cells in colostrum are white blood cells that guard against infections, helping your baby start fighting infections for themselves.

Everyone's milk comes in at different times depending on the type of birth you had and what number baby this is for you. If you had a cesarean birth, you might see it come in between days four and six, whereas if you had an unmedicated vaginal birth or have already had a baby, you may see it come in as early as day two. Keep your baby at the breast as much as possible; this stimulation tells your pituitary gland that baby is here and it's time to make milk. If you're concerned about your milk coming in, consult a lactation specialist.

Q. My baby is losing weight. Should I be worried?

It is normal for a baby to lose up to 10 percent of their birth weight with the expectation that they are back to their birth weight by two weeks. Remember, babies are born full of meconium, so when they pass meconium, they will lose weight. There is also the understanding that both you and baby are learning how to breastfeed the first couple of weeks, so we expect some speed bumps before you find your rhythm. By two weeks, most problems are typically resolved or improving, and baby should start gaining weight. If not, you can look into supplementing with donor breast milk or formula; a lactation specialist can help you supplement at the breast so that there is stimulation, signaling your breasts to make milk.

Q. My breasts are huge and painful. How do I treat engorgement?

Engorgement feels like you woke up with breast implants three sizes too big for the skin on your chest, and sometimes this can hurt like crazy. The most important thing to remember is that stimulation signals to the body that it needs to make more milk, so while pumping to drain the milk might seem like the right thing to do, this will actually increase milk production. Instead, try to nurse as much as possible. If they are too full, causing your nipple to be flat where baby can't latch, get in a warm shower and hand express, letting the milk drip out in there. If none of these things is working and your breast just won't drain, you can try a breast pump for three to five minutes to soften the breast slightly so baby can attempt to nurse. There is also a product on the market called the Haakaa silicone breast pump, which suctions onto the nipple and allows the breast to drain without stimulation. A similar product, called the Milkies Milk-Saver, will collect milk from the non-nursing side while you nurse on the other side, and this can help ease engorgement if baby isn't getting to both sides in one feeding. You can also use raw green cabbage to reduce the swelling. There is a natural enzyme in cabbage that helps with swelling and engorgement, so placing cabbage leaves in your bra may help.

Q. How do I breastfeed my baby? How do I know if I'm doing it right and my baby is getting enough to eat?

There's no way I can teach you how to breastfeed your baby in such a short amount of space! But I can point you in the right direction. To start, find a breastfeeding class or talk to a lactation consultant prior to giving birth. This will give you a general overview of how to breastfeed and connect you to all of the resources in your area. If you can't find a breastfeeding class, connect with your local La Leche League group (llli.org/get-help). A lactation consultant or breastfeeding class will be able to show you latching techniques, common nursing positions that will help ease the process, and ways to learn your baby's hunger signs.

Lactation support from knowledgeable teachers and other moms who are going through or have been through what you're going through is also an invaluable tool, especially in those early nursing days—you can find this through a La Leche League meeting. There are also amazing online resources where you can get visuals of what a proper latch looks like along with different ways to position your baby. We have a helpful free guide which can be found at TheBirth-Hour.com/breastfeeding.

Be sure to have breastfeeding stations around your house, as most of your time will be spent nursing. These stations should include your nursing pillow, water, breast pads or the Milkies Milk-Saver (to catch leaking milk on the non-nursing side), nipple ointment, a snack, and something like a book to help you pass the time.

Q. Help! Breastfeeding hurts. Should it feel this way? What can I do to fix it?

The first week of breastfeeding typically comes with some pain, especially when baby first latches on. You will read that if your nipples hurt, you aren't doing it right. There are many factors that come into play plus the whole learning curve associated with both of you figuring out your nursing relationship; as such, there might be pain from time to time. Another issue that may come up is your baby having a tongue and/or lip tie, which can drastically affect how the baby latches, sucks, and swallows milk. This can be evaluated by a lactation professional and revised by a pediatric dentist. The bottom line is: If you're having painful feeds, be sure to seek help in person. Have your latch assessed and baby's mouth assessed, and gather all the pointers that can help clear up any problems. It will not be like this forever, and you're not alone in this process. Breastfeeding can be really challenging for the first few weeks, but by about week three or four, you will hopefully have found your rhythm.

Q. I have inverted or flat nipples. Can I still breastfeed?

Yes! Right now, suck on the side of your hand. There's no nipple and it's a flat surface, but if you suck you will create suction and be able to draw something into your mouth. It's the same with your breasts and flat or inverted nipples. Your baby will be able to draw the tissue into their mouth and express milk. In some cases, using a pump for a minute before latching draws the nipple out and can be helpful. In other cases, nipple shields might be recommended. If you're concerned, see a lactation specialist and have them assess what might work best for you.

Q. How can I tell if I have clogged ducts or mastitis? What can I do to prevent this from happening? And what can I do to treat it?

It is typically very easy to tell if you have a clogged duct or mastitis because it is quite painful. There may be a visible red area on the breast, and it's likely very tender to touch. With a clogged duct, the most important thing to do is massage it frequently to try to break up the clog. You can use massage oil and massage toward the nipple. Even though this might be painful, it will help your situation. If the clogged duct turns into mastitis, it is usually accompanied by a fever and flu-like symptoms. Talk to your care provider; you will likely be prescribed antibiotics. Essential oils, green cabbage leaves, and ultrasound technology can also be used on both a clog and mastitis to help heal and break up the infection. Seek professional help from a lactation specialist immediately if you're dealing with these issues.

Q. How can I tell if my baby has a tongue or lip tie? What can be done to fix it?

Tongue and lip ties are very common, and they can affect breast-feeding. The problem is that most providers haven't caught up with current research regarding this problem. The best way for your baby to be assessed is to ask your lactation specialist or pediatrician if they have experience with tongue and lip ties. If they don't, ask for recommendations. Most practitioners use the HATLFF assessment tool by Elizabeth Hazelbaker to assess tongue and lip ties. Many pediatric dentists now specialize in revising these ties using cold CO_2 lasers.

Q. How can I manage a forceful letdown or oversupply?

This is a very common problem, especially in the beginning of nursing, because there seems to be an overabundance of milk in the first few weeks. The most important thing is not to pump for an oversupply because that signals your body to make more milk. For a forceful letdown, it can be helpful to pump for two minutes before nursing your baby so your pump gets the first letdown and the rest of your feeding should be a lot less forceful. Milk supply typically regulates by about six weeks. If it doesn't, it's still a variation of normal, and a lactation specialist can assist with other techniques by observing baby's latch and feeding.

Q. How do I know if I have a low milk supply? Should I supplement?

The goal is for your baby to be back to birth weight by two weeks. If you're having problems with your baby gaining weight, be sure to see a lactation specialist immediately. They will diagnose what's going on and help you make adjustments to increase your supply. If you can't find a lactation specialist in your area, be sure to ask your pediatrician. In terms of supplementing, this is a conversation to have with your pediatrician. Be sure they are breastfeeding-friendly if that's something you feel strongly about.

Q. What can I do to increase my milk supply?

There are several natural methods to increase your milk supply. The first is making sure that you have a good latch and that baby is effective at sucking and emptying your breast. Once that has been assessed, many lactation experts will start with a galactagogue (a milk-stimulating substance), such as fenugreek, moringa fennel, or goat's rue. These can be taken as tinctures or pills and are sometimes baked into cookies. Increasing the stimulation to the breast will trigger your pituitary gland to make more milk as well, so nurse frequently. Get in touch with a lactation specialist to see what methods will help you best.

Q. What is donor milk, and how do I get it?

There are several companies across the nation that sell pasteurized breast milk to NICUs. In recent years, there has been an influx of social media groups that are increasing access to donor milk through donors with an overabundance of milk along with safer milk-sharing practices. The most popular one, Eats on Feets (eatsonfeets.org/ #resource, also on Facebook), created the following list, "The 4 Pillars of Safe Milk Sharing."

Informed choice
» Understanding the options, including the risks and benefits, of all infant and child feeding methods
» Know thy source

Donor screening
» Donor self-exclusion for or declaration of medical and social concerns
» Communication about lifestyle and habits
» Screening for HIV I and II, HTLV I and II, HBV, HCV, syphilis, and rubella

Safe handling

» Inspecting and keeping skin, hands, and equipment clean

» Properly handling, storing, transporting, and shipping breast milk

Home pasteurization

» Heat-treating milk to address infectious pathogens

» Informed choice of raw milk when donor criteria are met

» Another popular resource is Human Milk for Human Babies

Another good way to obtain milk is through asking in your friend circle. There may be people who have an oversupply. Just be sure to follow the safe milk sharing practices.

Q. Can I drink coffee and alcohol while breastfeeding?

Good question! The answer: Everything in moderation, just as in pregnancy. These substances do pass through to your breast milk. In terms of coffee, the same rule goes as in pregnancy; around eight to 12 ounces of caffeinated beverages is okay while nursing. With alcohol, the common recommendation is that the occasional glass of wine, beer, or a cocktail will not affect your baby. However, if you go out for a night on the town and consume more than that, it's recommended to pump and dump your milk. The general rule of thumb is that if it smells like alcohol or if you have consumed enough that you are impaired by alcohol, it isn't safe to nurse your baby.

Q. How do I know what medications I can take while breastfeeding?

Since the early 1990s, Dr. Thomas Hale has been setting the gold standard regarding medications and breast milk. His database is constantly updated, and this is the best resource to find out if a medication is safe for use during lactation (HalesMeds.com). Each medication is given a classification in a rating system, with L1 being the safest and L5 being contraindicated. Even some doctors aren't aware of this resource, so it's okay to advocate for yourself when picking a medication. Another great resource is KellyMom.com.

Q. My baby is spitting up constantly. Should I be concerned?

Keep in mind that what seems like a ton of spit-up to you—because it soaked you and baby—is likely just a tablespoon or so. While some spit-up is normal and typically goes away when baby starts sitting on their own, it can be annoying and makes some babies very fussy. If this is the case for you, chiropractic care or cranio-sacral therapy can be useful to try to correct this problem. If there's no relief and you're worried, be sure to check with your pediatrician to rule out reflux issues.

"Pregnancy complications can make you a better mother. We chose to be thankful for every day of pregnancy, birth, the NICU stay, and beyond. We know what it's like to be told 'your baby will most likely not make it to birth.' We also know how strong you become when you choose to believe she will."

—Lexie Emory

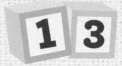

Pregnancy and Labor Complications

Dr. Emiliano Chavira, MD, MPH, FACOG

This book is designed to address questions related to normal, uncomplicated pregnancies and births. However, sometimes things come up during pregnancy that are unexpected or may change the way your care provider approaches your treatment or birth. In this chapter, Dr. Chavira will go over some of those things and offer advice for navigating the unexpected. As always, you should consult your care provider when any concerns arise.

Q. I'm vomiting all the time, and my doctor mentioned hyperemesis gravidarum. What can I expect if I have HG?

Nausea and vomiting are extremely common in early pregnancy. Hyperemesis, however, is a severe form of nausea and vomiting that can result in weight loss, electrolyte abnormalities (sodium, potassium, etc.), and hospitalization. The line between ordinary nausea and vomiting of pregnancy and hyperemesis is a bit fuzzy, but it's generally considered hyperemesis if you need IV fluids or lose over 5 percent of your original weight. If you have hyperemesis, you will need to eat small meals or bites of food continuously throughout the day and take small sips of whatever you can keep down to stay hydrated. Avoid things that trigger your nausea. You may try various therapies like acupuncture, magnetic bracelets, and ginger (ginger ale, tea, essential oil, candies, capsules, etc.), but your care provider will likely need to prescribe medications for you. You may have to try a few different medications or combinations before finding the right one. Dehydration can cause your nausea and vomiting to get worse. In these cases, you will need to go to the hospital for blood work, IV fluids, and anti-nausea medications. If you have hyperemesis gravidarum, you may end up visiting the hospital more than once for varying lengths of time. For most pregnancies, these symptoms will get much better or even go away completely somewhere between 16 and 20 weeks, but sometimes they continue throughout the pregnancy. One thing to know is that if the hyperemesis goes away, it will not come back. This is important because if the nausea and vomiting go away and then come back at a later time, they should no longer be considered hyperemesis. In this case your care provider needs to look for an alternative explanation for the nausea and vomiting.

Q. What are the symptoms of an ectopic pregnancy, and how is it treated?

An ectopic pregnancy is a pregnancy that implants and starts growing somewhere in the body outside the uterus. The most common location for ectopic pregnancies is in one of the fallopian tubes, although they can be found in other places. Very early on, an ectopic pregnancy may feel like any other pregnancy, with symptoms like nausea, vomiting, and breast tenderness. At some point, you will begin to have some vaginal bleeding. As the pregnancy begins stretching and perhaps even tearing the fallopian tube, there will usually be abdominal pain below the belly button, usually on one side or the other. Based on the pregnancy's progression, you may also feel dizzy or light-headed, and you may begin to feel some pain in your shoulders caused by blood in the abdominal cavity. An ectopic pregnancy is diagnosed by blood tests and ultrasound. In some cases, they are detected on an ultrasound before any major symptoms develop, but they are most often diagnosed during evaluation of lower abdominal pain and vaginal bleeding.

Ectopic pregnancies must be treated because in most cases they will rupture and cause internal bleeding, which puts your life in danger. An ectopic pregnancy cannot be moved into the uterus and cannot be saved. Ectopic pregnancies can be terminated medically with an injection of methotrexate or via surgery. When methotrexate is given, your care provider will monitor you closely over the following days to ensure that the injection worked. Surgical removal can be done with an open incision or with laparoscopy, which involves passing a camera and instruments through small incisions on your belly. In some cases, but not all, the entire fallopian tube is removed with the ectopic pregnancy inside it. If only the ectopic pregnancy is removed and the fallopian tube is left in place, then you will need to have a weekly pregnancy blood test to make sure that the ectopic pregnancy was completely removed.

Q. I was told I have a short cervix. How does this affect my pregnancy?

The cervix is the lowest part of the uterus, leading to the vagina. As the baby grows and the uterus expands, the cervix is supposed to remain long and closed and usually measures three to five centimeters long. A short cervix is when the cervical length is 2.5 centimeters or less. If the cervix is found to be short early in the pregnancy (between 16 and 24 weeks), there is a higher-than-normal risk of a preterm birth. A short cervix during the third trimester is not as significant as it is in the first half of the pregnancy. If your cervix is short, there are a few treatment options available that have been shown to reduce the chances of a preterm birth. One is vaginal progesterone, which is given by inserting a progesterone pill or suppository into the vagina every night. Another common option is a cervical cerclage, which is when a surgical suture is sewn around the cervix to help keep it closed. A newer option that is less commonly used is a pessary, which is a supportive device placed inside the vagina. Traditionally, bed rest was prescribed, but this recommendation has become outdated (see page 57), though some providers may still recommend it. Having a short cervix in a prior pregnancy doesn't automatically mean that you will have a short cervix again in a subsequent pregnancy. Keep in mind that a short cervix is just a risk factor. It does not mean for sure that you will have a preterm birth. It just means that your chances of delivering early are higher than average.

Q. What is pelvic-floor rest, and how will it affect my pregnancy?

Pelvic-floor rest means that nothing is inserted into the vagina. This means no tampons, no douching, and, of course, no intercourse. This advice is commonly given to women with certain pregnancy symptoms like first trimester bleeding, preterm labor, premature rupture of membranes, and placenta previa (when the placenta is low in the uterus and covering the cervix). There isn't a good base of studies to support the notion that pelvic rest actually makes the pregnancy safer. This advice is really just based on the fact that it may make sense in some cases. Miscarriage is very clearly *not* caused by physical activity, so pelvic rest for first trimester bleeding may not make sense. Nevertheless, many care providers continue to make this recommendation. On the other hand, pelvic rest does make sense in cases like premature rupture of membranes and placenta previa, especially if there has been bleeding.

Q. Does the positioning of my placenta affect my baby?

ANTERIOR VERSUS POSTERIOR

Whether the placenta is located anteriorly (attached to the front wall of the uterus) or posteriorly (attached to the back wall of the uterus) really makes no difference in most cases. Some people say it may take you longer to feel fetal movements if the placenta is anterior, but this concept is not backed up by studies and may just be an old wives' tale. An anterior placenta may be an issue of concern if you've ever had a surgical incision on either the front or back of the uterus; for example, for a prior cesarean or a myomectomy (surgery to remove one or more uterine myomas or fibroids from the uterus). If the placenta implants on the uterus over an existing uterine scar, there is a risk of developing a placenta accreta. Placenta accreta is discussed in more detail on the next page.

LOW-LYING PLACENTA

The definition of a low-lying placenta is when the lowest edge of the placenta is within two centimeters of the cervix but not covering it. In the vast majority of cases, the placenta will move upward during the course of the pregnancy, and very few placentas are still low-lying at term. If the placenta is still low-lying at term, there may be an increased risk of severe bleeding at the time of childbirth. Because of this, cesarean is often recommended when a placenta is low-lying at term, but this is something to discuss with your care provider.

PLACENTA PREVIA

Placenta previa is when the placenta is implanted so low in the uterus that it covers the cervix. Vaginal birth with a placenta previa would most likely result in massive hemorrhage in childbirth, so a cesarean is always recommended. The good news is that this situation usually corrects itself and there is no longer a previa once the pregnancy has gotten to term. This is especially likely to happen if only the edge of the placenta is covering the cervix as opposed to a central previa where the whole placenta is implanted right over the cervix. Sometimes, when a placenta previa is present, there may be episodes of vaginal bleeding during the pregnancy requiring hospitalization until the bleeding stops. This may happen more than once during the pregnancy. In rare cases, a cesarean delivery may need to occur prematurely due to serious bleeding.

PLACENTA ACCRETA

In a typical pregnancy, the placenta attaches itself to the uterine wall in a controlled fashion. The attachment is strong enough to be stable throughout the whole pregnancy, but the placenta is designed to detach from the uterus and come out at the time of childbirth. Placenta accreta means that the placenta has attached too deeply into (or through) the uterine wall. In these cases, the placenta will not detach from the uterus at the time of birth, putting the birthing person's life in serious danger. When a placenta accreta is present, the delivery is accomplished by performing a cesarean. However, after the baby has been delivered, the uterus itself is removed with the placenta still inside it. The uterine cervix may or may not also be removed as part of the surgery. This procedure is called cesarean hysterectomy. The risks of a cesarean hysterectomy are much higher than the risks of a routine cesarean. Most cases involve several liters of blood loss, meaning blood transfusions are required. Those who undergo a cesarean hysterectomy are often admitted to the ICU until they have stabilized from this major surgery. Although placenta accreta can happen in any pregnancy, it is extremely rare if there have been no prior uterine surgeries. The most common situation in which placenta accreta happens is when there is a history of one or more cesareans and the placenta implants over the cesarean scar. The higher the number of prior cesareans, the higher the chances of having a placenta accreta. An accreta can also develop when there is a history of uterine myomectomy or even D&C, but this is much less common. The best way to avoid the problem of placenta accreta is to avoid having that first cesarean, if possible.

Q. If I'm considered "high risk," how will that affect my pregnancy and birth?

As mentioned on page 24, the term "high risk" is overused and applied to many situations in which the risk of certain complications is only very slightly higher than the average population risk. A pregnancy being labeled "high risk" doesn't mean you will encounter any major complications. There are myriad reasons why you may be considered high risk, such as age, a history of preterm birth, and carrying multiples; treatments are based on each condition with some requiring nothing more than additional testing or frequent monitoring. In other, more severe cases, your care provider may work with a perinatologist or refer you to their care for the remainder of your pregnancy (see page 22).

Sometimes if you have had a prior cesarean, you are considered high risk. However, in most cases you should have a choice between a vaginal birth after cesarean (VBAC) or a planned repeat cesarean birth, but many doctors don't support VBAC, and some hospitals even have explicit policies against VBAC. If you wish to have a VBAC, you may have to work hard to find a supportive doctor and hospital. The International Cesarean Awareness Network (ICAN) is a great resource, as most cities have a local chapter where you can ask for recommendations.

Some multiple gestations (pregnancies with more than one baby) have higher risks than others and will likely require more ultrasounds compared to women carrying one baby. Multiple gestations can deliver vaginally, and studies show that this is just as safe as a cesarean. Unfortunately, it is becoming increasingly common for doctors to recommend cesarean delivery for twins (or higher multiples) even though the studies do not support this practice, so this is an important conversation to have with your care provider.

Sometimes pregnancies are considered high risk because of a birth defect or other problem in the baby. While a handful of these conditions can be treated during the pregnancy, there may not be any treatments available until after the baby is born. These births typically happen in larger hospitals where the necessary pediatric specialists are available. For information about the specific tests that may be necessary in the late stages of pregnancy, see page 31.

Q. I'm over the age of 35. What do I need to know about advanced maternal age and pregnancy?

Advanced maternal age is associated with greater chances of having a baby with certain genetic conditions, like Down syndrome. There are several testing options to evaluate this if you so desire. Apart from the genetic testing question, prenatal care is essentially the same as for anyone else. There is a slightly higher chance of developing certain complications in pregnancy, like gestational diabetes or preeclampsia, and there is also a statistically higher chance of having a cesarean birth. Some care providers might recommend delivering the baby a little earlier than normal, like 40 or even 39 weeks, but this is not a universal practice. If you're over the age of 35, you may be wondering if your body can tolerate a vaginal birth. There is no reason to think that it can't, and there is no reason to plan a cesarean birth simply on the basis of your age.

Q. I'm having twins! How will my pregnancy differ from a singleton pregnancy?

All of the symptoms of pregnancy, such as nausea and vomiting or aches and pains, may be exaggerated in a twin pregnancy due to higher levels of hCG (human chorionic gonadotropin, a hormone that the placenta produces). Some twin pregnancies have two placentas (dichorionic twin gestation), in which each twin is attached to its very own placenta. Dichorionic twin pregnancies are often called "high risk," but the reality is that the risk is not dramatically different than a singleton pregnancy. Prenatal care is also essentially the same for a dichorionic twin pregnancy.

In contrast, there are other twin pregnancies in which both twins are attached to and share the same placenta (monochorionic twin gestation). These pregnancies can have special complications due to the fact that the twins are sharing one placenta and also that their umbilical cord blood supplies are connected within the placenta. These pregnancies are usually monitored much more closely with ultrasound exams every two weeks starting at 16 weeks' gestation. These exams are typically performed by a perinatologist unless the OB is very experienced in caring for twins. Whether a twin pregnancy can be cared for by a midwife depends on state law.

Q. What are my childbirth options with twins?

Twins can be delivered vaginally or by cesarean. Several twin studies in recent years have shown that vaginal birth is at least as safe or even safer than cesarean birth. Despite this scientific evidence, doctors are increasingly recommending cesareans for twins. Unfortunately, the skills needed for twin vaginal birth are gradually decreasing among OBs. That said, some doctors do offer vaginal birth for twins, although their individual guidelines may vary from one to another and are dependent upon the position the babies are in before delivery, that is, head-down or breech. Very few doctors will offer a vaginal birth if the first twin is in a breech position, but there are a handful across the country who have these skills. Some doctors won't offer vaginal birth at all and may insist that you deliver by cesarean. If you're carrying a twin pregnancy and want to have a vaginal birth, you may have to work hard to find a provider who has maintained their twin vaginal birth skills and you will almost always be required to give birth in the OR just in case a cesarean is required. Some midwives are very experienced with twin vaginal birth, but again this will vary depending on state law regarding whether they can attend your twin birth.

Q. I have gestational diabetes. How is it treated?

The first line of treatment is a diabetic diet, which is low in carbohydrates and sugars, and regular exercise. Usually, diet and exercise are enough to keep the blood sugar levels normal. You will also likely be checking your own blood sugar four times per day and keeping a log of your numbers. If your blood sugar is normal with diet and exercise, then you will continue that regime. If your blood sugar is persistently high even with improved diet and exercise, then medications are used to help keep your blood sugar at a normal level. There are oral medications that can be used, and there is also insulin, which is injected. Insulin is generally considered to be the best treatment in cases where medication is needed. High levels of sugar in your bloodstream pass into your baby's bloodstream, which can have a harmful effect on your baby, so it is critically important to keep your blood sugar at normal levels not only for your health but for your baby's well-being as well.

Q. What is preeclampsia, and what does it mean for my baby and me?

Preeclampsia is a condition marked primarily by high blood pressure in the second half of pregnancy. Although it can happen any time after 20 weeks, most cases happen closer to the end of the pregnancy, are mild, and are not dangerous for either you or your baby. However, preeclampsia may get worse as time passes, and any case can progress into a severe form that can be quite dangerous for both mother and baby. If needed, medications can be given to keep the blood pressure from rising to dangerously high levels. However, even if the blood pressure is temporarily controlled, the preeclampsia is still there and can continue to get worse over time.

The only way to cure preeclampsia is to deliver the baby, thus ending the pregnancy. If preeclampsia appears after 37 weeks, the usual recommendation is to proceed with delivery, either by induction or cesarean. This recommendation is based on the idea that the baby is sufficiently mature to be born, so it isn't worthwhile to continue the pregnancy and risk the preeclampsia progressing to the point where it could harm you, your baby, or both of you. On the other hand, if preeclampsia appears earlier than 37 weeks, it might be desirable to try to extend the pregnancy to allow the baby to mature as much as possible before proceeding with delivery. In general, if the preeclampsia is mild and remains mild, you and baby will be monitored closely with the goal of delaying delivery until 37 weeks, if possible.

Q. What is intrauterine growth restriction (IUGR)?

Intrauterine growth restriction, or IUGR, refers to a situation in which the baby is thought to be smaller than expected for a given gestational age. There is some degree of inaccuracy to this diagnosis because ultrasound estimations of fetal weight are known to have a built-in error rate. Also, growing babies normally come in a wide range of sizes, and some are just naturally small. At term, a baby might weigh six pounds or 11 pounds, and both may be normal! A commonly agreed-upon definition of growth restriction is when the estimated fetal weight is under the 10th percentile, but many of those babies will actually be healthy and growing normally. However, if a baby measures below a lower cutoff, like fifth percentile or third percentile, the chances are higher that the baby may truly be growth restricted. IUGR can be seen in cases where the baby has some kind of health condition, like a genetic disorder or a serious infection. In other cases, the problem lies in the placenta. The placenta might not be working at full capacity and therefore may not be supporting the baby completely, and the baby grows less as a consequence. When IUGR is diagnosed, those pregnancies are monitored more intensively than uncomplicated pregnancies. NSTs are usually performed twice per week (see page 31). There may also be specialized ultrasound exams that look at the circulation through the placenta and the baby's body. Unfortunately, there are no medications that can be given to make the placenta work better or to help the baby grow normally. Also, when IUGR is present, there is a slightly higher risk of stillbirth. Because of this, it may be advisable to deliver the baby a little earlier than usual, like 37 to 39 weeks. In very severe cases of IUGR, delivery may even be recommended as early as 32 to 34 weeks.

Q. My baby is breech. How do I get it to turn head down?

Babies are very commonly in a breech position (bottom-down instead of head-down) early in the pregnancy. They have a lot of freedom to move and change positions frequently. Because of this, if your baby is in a breech presentation in the second trimester, you shouldn't worry about it. Most babies will get into a head-down position on their own by the time the pregnancy reaches term. Only about 3 percent of babies will still be breech by this time. If you get to about 34 weeks and the baby is still breech, there are some things you can try to help your baby turn into a head-down position. Prior to starting any of these treatments, you should have an ultrasound to see if any specific cause for the breech presentation can be found, such as placenta previa, large uterine fibroid tumors blocking the birth canal, or major structural birth defects in the baby. Trying to get the baby into a head-down position only makes sense if vaginal birth is possible in the first place, and it usually is in most cases.

FORWARD-LEANING INVERSIONS AND BREECH TILT EXERCISES

These exercises involve turning yourself almost upside down several times per day to help the baby flip. They are described in more detail on the Spinning Babies website (SpinningBabies.com).

CHIROPRACTIC CARE

Some chiropractors offer an adjustment called the Webster Technique, which works on the pelvis and round ligaments of the uterus. This has been reported to help some babies turn to a head-down position, although there are few studies published in medical literature regarding how effective this technique is. Some chiropractors say that even if the baby does not turn with the Webster Technique, it may help increase the effectiveness of an external cephalic version (ECV) procedure (see below).

EASTERN MEDICINE

There are a few techniques derived from Eastern medicine that have been described as helpful for turning breech babies. Acupuncture has been employed to help turn breech babies. Another treatment is moxibustion, in which an herbal moxa stick is burned and held to your toe. It has also been suggested that holding something cold at the top of the uterus (like a bag of frozen peas) may stimulate the baby to move to a head-down position. Again, the studies that have attempted to test these treatments to see how well they work are limited. However, they are unlikely to be harmful and therefore may be worth a try.

EXTERNAL CEPHALIC VERSION (ECV)

This is a procedure in which a doctor or other provider places their hands on your belly and tries to push the baby around into a head-down position. This option is usually considered if you get to 37 weeks and none of the other therapies have helped the baby to flip. There are many studies on ECV. Published success rates tend to run around 50 to 60 percent, although success rates are lower in the first pregnancy and higher for those who have previously given birth. The success rate of ECV procedures can be increased by using uterine-relaxing medications (especially terbutaline) and epidural anesthesia. Because the ECV has a low risk of complications and has been shown to reduce the chances of having a cesarean, the American College of Obstetricians and Gynecologists (ACOG) recommends that all pregnant people with a breech baby near term be offered an ECV unless it would be inappropriate for some specific reason, like placenta previa.

Q. If my baby is still breech when my due date arrives, what are my options for childbirth?

If your baby is still breech as the due date approaches, you can try any of the approaches discussed in the previous question if you have not yet done so. But if it appears that your baby is determined to stay in a breech position or if you would prefer not to try to turn the baby, then there are two options for your birth. One is to plan for vaginal birth, and the other is to plan for cesarean birth. In the United States, very few doctors have the skills and willingness to participate in a breech vaginal birth. Therefore, if you're under the care of a doctor, a cesarean will almost always be recommended. This is an extremely difficult circumstance for those women who have a strong desire to avoid cesarean, but it is unfortunately the current reality.

If you're under the care of a midwife, you're more likely to be offered a vaginal birth, as some midwives (but not all) are highly experienced in attending breech births. Whether your midwife can offer you a planned vaginal birth will depend on state law and the experience of that particular midwife. There are a large number of studies suggesting that vaginal breech birth is safe in the presence of a skilled breech provider. That said, all breech birth experts agree that a vaginal breech birth is more likely to become complicated than a head-down birth, so it is only advisable to attempt a breech birth when a knowledgeable and experienced breech provider is with you. More information can be found at InformedPregnancy.com/heads-up.

If cesarean birth is planned, there are two ways to do this. The first is to schedule the cesarean for a specific date, like 39 weeks, for example. This approach allows you to choose the birthday to some degree. The second is to wait for labor to start and then do the cesarean on that day. This approach allows the baby to choose the birth date.

Q. What are the main causes and symptoms of preterm labor?

Preterm labor is caused by a wide variety of factors. Some common causes are inflammation in the uterine cavity caused by microorganisms, bleeding behind the placenta, or premature rupture of the membranes. Genetics may also be a factor. Multiple gestation pregnancies are more likely to deliver preterm compared to singletons. Intense emotional or physiological stress can also lead to preterm birth. Severe emotional stress could include things like a divorce, losing a job, or a death in the family, whereas physiological stress might be something like starvation, severe illness, or drug abuse. Black women are known to have higher rates of preterm birth than other women, and it is being increasingly recognized that much of this is caused by the chronic stress that comes from living in a society permeated with racism as well as the unequal treatment they receive in medical institutions like hospitals.

Symptoms of preterm labor are the same symptoms that occur with labor at term, the most common being uterine contractions. Contractions cause a crampy pain similar to menstrual cramps. They come on and then pass like a wave, lasting one to two minutes. During a contraction, you may notice that your uterus feels hard. You may feel pain in the lower part of your belly or in your lower back. Contractions that occur a few times per day with no particular rhythm are not likely to be a problem. On the other hand, if the contractions start to have a rhythm—for example, every 10 minutes or every five minutes—then this might be a sign of preterm labor. It is especially concerning if the contractions begin to get stronger and closer together over time. If your cervix is shortening or dilating, you might notice an increase in vaginal discharge, spotting, or even bleeding. Leaking fluid from your vagina could mean that the bag of water has popped or is leaking. If any of these symptoms occur, you should contact your care provider right away or go to the hospital for evaluation.

Q. Are there ways to prevent or stop preterm labor?

One approach to prevent preterm labor is to get as healthy as possible before getting pregnant. Focus on healthy food choices, hydration, and regular exercise. If you're a smoker, start cutting down or, better yet, quit altogether before getting pregnant. If you have medical issues like diabetes, high blood pressure, or thyroid problems, see your regular doctor and make sure these conditions are well controlled before proceeding with pregnancy. If you're already pregnant, it's never too late to start developing healthy habits. Many people think it's important to minimize physical activity in pregnancy, but in fact the opposite is true. Research has shown that women who exercise in pregnancy have better outcomes, and restriction of physical activity in a couple of studies has even been associated with *increased* rates of preterm birth.

Try to get a good night's sleep as often as possible. Start the day off with a nutritious breakfast, as prolonged fasting is a physiological stressor in pregnancy. Stress is an unavoidable part of modern life, but try to control it as much as possible. Practicing mindfulness, regular meditation, or even yoga may help.

From a medical point of view, ultrasound examination of the cervix in mid-pregnancy may be helpful. Some centers routinely perform an ultrasound exam of the cervix as part of prenatal care, while other centers do this only if there are risk factors for preterm birth. If the cervix is found to be short, there are various treatments that can be offered (see page 169). These treatments are not helpful if the cervical length is normal.

All of these approaches focus on prevention of preterm birth before any symptoms develop. If true preterm labor begins at some point in the pregnancy, there is probably no way to stop it. There are several medications that can slow contractions temporarily, but there are hundreds of studies that have essentially shown that once preterm labor starts, it cannot effectively be stopped. However, there are some things that can be done to help a baby who is about to be born prematurely. To begin with, you might be moved to a hospital that has a NICU capable of caring for a premature baby if there is time to do so. Corticosteroid injections are given to help baby's lungs develop and substantially reduce breathing complications after birth. If you deliver before 32 weeks, magnesium, which has been shown to reduce the chances of your baby developing cerebral palsy (a disorder of coordination and movement), will be administered. Finally, antibiotics may be given since preemies are more susceptible and more vulnerable to infections. Medical science has not yet found an effective way to stop preterm labor once it has begun, but the treatment of preemie babies has improved, and they now have much better survival rates and better outcomes than they did even a few decades ago.

Q. Why is my doctor worried about my baby being too big?

Obstetric providers as a whole tend to be very worried about the possibility of a "big baby." The main reason behind this high level of concern is the fear of a difficult and even traumatic childbirth (meaning severe injury to you or your baby). The bigger the baby is, the higher the risk of a traumatic birth. On the one hand, there are births where injuries occur, and some can be devastating or even fatal. However, the level of concern is often blown out of proportion compared to the actual risk. The medical term for "big baby" is macrosomia. Studies of birth outcomes for macrosomic babies show that the risk of severe injury in childbirth is much lower than you might expect, but some care providers commonly raise concerns about suspected macrosomia. This can be a problem because unhelpful recommendations are often given, such as induction of labor "to prevent the baby from getting too big." This does not mean that continuing to wait for natural labor has no risk. There is always a small risk of serious trauma in childbirth. But if labor is induced, the risk of birth trauma is *the same*, not less. The ACOG has said in its published guidelines that induction of labor for suspected macrosomia does not improve outcomes for mothers or their babies.

Another common scenario is to receive a recommendation to have a cesarean because vaginal birth, in the opinion of the care provider, would be too dangerous. Estimates of fetal weight by ultrasound are known to be inaccurate, and labor and delivery units across the country deliver babies by cesarean because they are thought to be too big only to find the babies to be one or two pounds *less* than the ultrasound estimate. Even if the estimated fetal weight was exactly correct, most of these births will not be traumatic. Many can deliver nine-, 10-, and even 11-pound babies without any serious complications. But if all "big babies" are delivered by cesarean, then many birthgivers will have cesareans when they could have had uncomplicated vaginal births. Finally, delivery by cesarean is not a "zero risk" alternative to vaginal birth. Surgery has plenty of risks of its own, both in the current pregnancy and in future pregnancies. In rare cases, complications from cesarean can be very serious and even fatal. The ACOG does not recommend cesarean based on estimated fetal size. It does say that cesarean "may be considered" if the estimated fetal weight is above five kilograms in a non-diabetic pregnancy. Evidence Based Birth (EvidenceBasedBirth.com) has an excellent article that reviews studies on "big babies" in detail.

Q. I have low amniotic fluid. What does this mean?

Historically, low amniotic fluid has been considered an important warning sign about the baby's health and has been used as a reason to deliver the baby in the hopes of preventing a stillbirth. However, this concern originally came from old, poorly designed studies that suggested a relationship between low fluid and stillbirth. Recent studies that have been careful to analyze only babies who have no apparent birth defects have not consistently found low fluid to be associated with stillbirth, meaning it's possible that low fluid is not as dangerous as we thought in the past. Still, this old idea that low fluid is dangerous continues to live on in modern obstetrics.

There are different ways of measuring amniotic fluid, and these methods often can lead to mixed messages and confusion. The older method is called AFI, for amniotic fluid index. The fluid is measured with ultrasound in the four corners of your belly, and these four numbers are added up. If the total number is less than five, this is considered low fluid, or oligohydramnios. The other way of measuring fluid is the deepest vertical pocket method. In this method, all pockets of fluid throughout the uterus are looked at with ultrasound, and the deepest one is measured. As long as this pocket is two centimeters deep or greater, then this is considered a normal fluid volume. Compared to the AFI method, the deepest vertical pocket method allows the fluid to fall to lower levels and still be considered normal. Studies comparing the two methods have shown fewer interventions using the deepest vertical pocket method, so this is the preferable method. If your fluid is found to be low by that method, then proceeding with delivery will likely be recommended.

Q. What is a post-term pregnancy, and is it safe to go past my due date?

In pregnancy, the word "term" means anything at 37 weeks or later. Term is further divided into several distinct periods. "Early term" is from 37 weeks to 38 weeks and six days. "Full term" is from 39 weeks to 40 weeks and six days. "Late term" is from 41 weeks to 41 weeks and six days. Finally, "post term" is anything from 42 weeks and beyond. In terms of safety, there is no magic point that divides the pregnancy into the categories of "safe" versus "unsafe." Even in a low-risk pregnancy, once you pass 39 weeks, the risk of stillbirth increases slightly week by week. The good news is that the risk is always low, no matter how many weeks you are. There are other risks besides stillbirth as the pregnancy goes further and further past the due date. One example is meconium aspiration syndrome, in which babies breathe meconium into their lungs; complications from this range from mild to a devastatingly severe illness in the newborn. The chance of having this complication also increases week by week; however, the overall risk is always low.

Because there are a small number of stillbirths and other complications in these last weeks of pregnancy, inducing labor in all birthing people at some chosen point will prevent a few stillbirths for a few birthing people. Preventing stillbirths is obviously a good thing, but there are some downsides to inducing labor, and the ACOG doesn't actually recommend inducing labor until 42 weeks. Despite this professional guideline, the reality is that most doctors recommend delivery sooner than this, commonly at 41 weeks. If you're comfortable inducing labor at the time that your care provider recommends, then it is reasonable to do so. On the other hand, if you have high hopes for an unmedicated birth that starts on its own, the risks of continuing the pregnancy and waiting for labor are pretty low. If you understand the risks of continuing the pregnancy and the risks of inducing labor, it is reasonable to make your own informed choice.

Q. What kind of labor complications would lead to a cesarean birth?

By far the most common reason for a cesarean in labor is arrested, or stalled, labor. This might mean that your cervix dilates up to a certain point but then doesn't dilate any further. Before six centimeters, dilation can be very slow, and it's important to be patient. After six centimeters, dilation should be continuous. The general guidelines say that we should wait at least four hours before diagnosing labor arrest, and in some cases it may be safe to wait even longer than that before deciding to have a C-section. Being patient helps to reduce the number of cesareans performed. Arrested labor can also happen after you're completely dilated. You may push for a number of hours, but the baby does not move down the birth canal. This type of labor arrest is called arrest of descent. Concerns about the fetal heart rate may also lead to a cesarean. Doctors vary widely in terms of how they respond to changes in fetal heart rate tracing. Some doctors will recommend a cesarean with minor abnormalities in the fetal heart rate tracing, whereas others will observe minor abnormalities carefully but allow the labor to continue.

The baby's position in labor can also require a cesarean. If the baby is found lying in a side-to-side orientation (this is called transverse) instead of head-down and cannot be repositioned, you may need a cesarean. A cord prolapse (when the umbilical cord falls out of the uterus ahead of the baby) will likely require a very quick emergency cesarean. If a high fever develops in labor, antibiotics are usually started, and your progress will be monitored closely. A cesarean may also become necessary in cases of preeclampsia, especially if the birth is not expected to happen within a short time frame. There is a condition known as placental abruption, in which the placenta begins to detach prematurely from the uterine wall. If it appears that an abruption is happening but both you and baby appear to be in good condition, labor can continue and often the baby can be born vaginally. However, if the abruption gets worse and either you or baby become unstable, then this may require an emergency cesarean. Some STIs, like genital herpes, can be another reason for an unexpected C-section. Most of the time, this diagnosis does not require a C-section, but if there's a herpes outbreak on the vulva at the time of labor, then the risk of passing the infection to the baby is higher, so a cesarean is recommended.

Q. What do I need to know about postpartum hemorrhaging?

Postpartum hemorrhage means heavy bleeding after birth. The current definition is simply a liter or more of blood lost in any birth or any blood loss that causes signs or symptoms in the birthing person. This is an important issue because, on a worldwide scale, postpartum hemorrhage accounts for about 10 percent of maternal deaths. In recent years, much attention has been paid to reducing maternal deaths from postpartum hemorrhage. If you're having heavy bleeding and you hear the term "postpartum hemorrhage," *do not panic*. Understand that postpartum hemorrhage is actually pretty common, and it is managed successfully in the vast majority of cases. Treatments will move quickly and may include medications to help the uterus contract, repair of a vaginal tear that may be bleeding, or insertion of a special balloon that is inflated inside the uterus to help control bleeding. If these kinds of measures are not controlling the bleeding, it may be necessary to perform surgery. If nothing is working, it may be necessary to perform a hysterectomy, which means complete removal of the uterus. In some cases, a uterine artery embolization may be used. A radiologist will insert a catheter into your pelvic arteries through a small puncture in the groin and inject a special material into the arteries leading to the uterus. This temporarily plugs those arteries to reduce blood flow to the uterus. You will likely need a blood transfusion as part of your treatment for severe postpartum hemorrhage. For women who will not accept transfusion on religious grounds, it is critical to be very aggressive about controlling bleeding as quickly as possible. If this is your case, discuss with your doctor ahead of time what products or procedures you are or are not willing to accept.

During pregnancy, if you're found to have anemia (low red cell count), work hard at getting your blood count up. See page 61 for information about treating low iron during pregnancy. At the time of childbirth, immediate and uninterrupted skin-to-skin contact between mother and baby is important for many reasons. Skin-to-skin contact triggers a massive release of oxytocin in the mother, which helps the uterus to contract down and stop bleeding. Breastfeeding is generally encouraged for many health benefits, and one of those benefits is that breastfeeding can help reduce your overall blood loss.

"Pregnancy loss is a life-changing event that brings feelings of grief, loneliness, and shame. Society makes it difficult for women and their partners to openly discuss this loss, which only magnifies its impact. Allow yourself to grieve, and don't hesitate to seek counseling to help you heal."

—Jennifer Carter

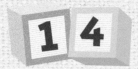

Pregnancy Loss

*Dr. Emiliano Chavira, MD, MPH, FACOG
and Courtney Butts, LMSW*

Unfortunately, loss is a necessary part of the
discussion around pregnancy. Hopefully
you will never need to reference this chapter.
However, the fact is that 10 to 20 percent of
recognized pregnancies end in loss, so you
likely know someone who has experienced
this. Typically, physical recovery from miscarriage happens quickly, but it may take much
longer to recover emotionally. In this chapter,
Dr. Chavira will answer questions related
to the physical aspects of miscarriage and
stillbirth, while Courtney Butts, our perinatal
mental health expert, will address the emotional and mental side of facing a loss.

Q. What is the difference between a chemical pregnancy and a miscarriage?

A chemical pregnancy is a very early miscarriage that happens before the pregnancy develops far enough to become visible on ultrasound. Both urine and blood pregnancy tests may give positive results, but nothing is ever seen on ultrasound. A chemical pregnancy is a real pregnancy, and it is a real miscarriage; it just happens very early on.

The term "miscarriage" refers to any pregnancy loss that happens before 20 weeks. Most miscarriages happen in the first few weeks of pregnancy, with the rate of miscarriage dropping to between 2 and 4 percent after week eight. By the end of the first trimester, the rate of miscarriage is less than 1 percent. While first trimester and second trimester losses are both types of miscarriage, they may have very different causes. First trimester miscarriages (less than 14 weeks) most often occur due to genetic abnormalities in the baby (see page 193 for more). Second trimester miscarriages (14 to 20 weeks) can be due to abnormalities in the baby but can also be caused by pregnancy complications like premature separation of the placenta or premature dilation of the cervix. If the baby passes away in utero in the second trimester, if abnormalities have been seen on ultrasound, or if genetic tests have suggested a problem, the cause of the second trimester miscarriage is likely to be a problem within the baby itself or its placenta. On the other hand, if the baby appears to be developing normally, the miscarriage might be attributable to a complication of pregnancy. For example, if you're having a lot of bleeding in the second trimester and it leads to miscarriage, this may be a placental abruption. In rare cases the uterine cervix may slowly dilate and lead to miscarriage, sometimes without any significant symptoms and without much warning. This is referred to in medical textbooks as painless cervical dilation.

Q. Do my chances of miscarriage go down as I get further along?

Yes, the further along you are, the lower the risk of miscarriage. The reason for this has to do with the reason why miscarriages happen in the first place. The most common cause of first trimester miscarriage (less than 14 weeks) is when the embryo, or early pregnancy, forms with genetic abnormalities. To be more specific, an egg and sperm each have 23 chromosomes (chromosomes contain the DNA, or genetic material, in each cell). When the egg and sperm fuse together during fertilization, this is supposed to create a single cell with 46 chromosomes, which is the normal number of chromosomes in humans. But the process of fertilization isn't always perfect. It's common for mistakes to happen during this fusion of cells, and the pregnancy can end up with missing or additional chromosomes. Pregnancies with the wrong number of chromosomes, in most cases, miscarry. Babies born with Down syndrome are one exception to this. A baby has Down syndrome when it forms with one extra copy of chromosome number 21 (for a total of 47 chromosomes). Many, but not all, pregnancies with Down syndrome will miscarry. Some babies with Down syndrome will survive the pregnancy and go on to live long lives. Why some Down syndrome babies miscarry and others don't isn't known.

Pregnancies that continue beyond the first trimester are much less likely to have chromosomal abnormalities, and because of this, they are much less likely to miscarry.

Q. Are miscarriages preventable?

Most first trimester miscarriages are not preventable. As discussed in the previous question, most miscarriages are caused by the embryo forming with the wrong number of chromosomes. However, there are some causes of miscarriage that *might* be preventable. Miscarriage is more common in the presence of certain medical conditions like uncontrolled diabetes or thyroid problems. There is a rare clotting disorder called antiphospholipid antibody syndrome that is also known to cause miscarriages and that is treated with blood thinners and aspirin. If you have diabetes, making sure that your blood sugar is very well controlled *before* you get pregnant will decrease your chances of having a miscarriage. The same might be said for thyroid conditions.

For many years, there has been a question about whether some miscarriages might be caused by low levels of a natural hormone called progesterone. This is challenging to study because it's hard to figure out if the low progesterone is a characteristic of the birthing person's physiology (which would therefore affect all of their pregnancies) or if it is a characteristic of the abnormal pregnancy itself (which would only be relevant to that particular pregnancy). There are some studies that support using progesterone treatment to reduce the chances of early miscarriage, especially for those with a history of prior miscarriages.

Smoking also increases the risk of miscarriage. If you use illegal drugs, avoiding them in pregnancy will reduce your chance of having a miscarriage. High levels of caffeine consumption have been associated with increased risk of miscarriage, so caffeine consumption should be limited.

It is also important to know that there are some things that very clearly *do not* cause miscarriage. Walking does not cause miscarriage. Running does not cause miscarriage. Exercise does not cause miscarriage. Having sex does not cause miscarriage. These are all healthy behaviors, and they are considered safe in pregnancy.

Q. I've had one or more miscarriages previously. What does this mean for my current pregnancy?

If you have had a *first trimester* miscarriage previously (less than 14 weeks), this should not make you worry about your current or future pregnancy. If you have had two or three miscarriages, you still have a high chance of having a successful pregnancy, but it might be worth looking into whether you have a condition that could be causing the miscarriages. Testing the pregnant person for diabetes and thyroid problems is standard. Both parents can have their chromosomes analyzed to see if one of the parents carries a chromosome that might be causing the miscarriages. If you have had three miscarriages or more, then testing for a rare clotting disorder called antiphospholipid antibody syndrome should be done. You should also have a pelvic exam and a pelvic ultrasound to look for any uterus malformations or masses, like uterine fibroids or myomas. In the past, it was standard to test for certain inherited clotting disorders like Factor V Leiden, Prothrombin G mutation, and MTHFR mutations, as older studies suggested a relationship between these conditions and recurrent miscarriage. However, newer, larger, and better-designed studies have shown that these conditions are not associated with miscarriage. Therefore, routine testing for these conditions is not currently recommended by the ACOG, but it is always your right to request extra tests and discuss your options with your care provider.

Remember that most first trimester miscarriages are due to genetic abnormalities in the baby, and therefore these miscarriages are really out of your hands. Of course, if a specific risk factor has been identified, then you can focus on making sure that condition is well controlled medically. See page 193 for more information on preventable miscarriages.

If you have had a prior *second trimester* miscarriage (14 to 20 weeks), this is a different issue. The details of your specific history are very important. If it seems that the problem was in the baby (abnormal ultrasound findings or abnormal genetic tests), then you don't need to worry if the current pregnancy seems to be developing normally. If your miscarriage was caused by an abruption, the chances that this will happen again are pretty low. Taking a low-dose aspirin once a day starting around 12 weeks might reduce the chances of having another abruption. If you suddenly delivered what appeared to be a normally developing baby and without much warning, then you may have had painless cervical dilation. The good news is that in most cases your next pregnancy will be uncomplicated, and this problem will not happen again. There are a couple of options when there is a history of second trimester miscarriage due to painless cervical dilation. See the sections on cervical cerclage and monitoring a short cervix (page 169) for more information.

Q. What are the chances of stillbirth, and can it be prevented?

Stillbirth refers to when a baby passes away while still inside the uterus, any time beyond 20 weeks' gestation. In pregnancies that pass 20 weeks, the chance of having a stillbirth is about six out of every 1,000 pregnancies. Some stillbirths might be preventable, but many are not since some are caused by underlying genetic conditions in the baby. Sometimes the specific diagnosis is known based on genetic testing. In such cases, the stillbirth might be expected or predictable to some degree but usually cannot be prevented. Some stillbirths happen suddenly in a pregnancy that appears to be developing normally. These cases are not preventable because there are no warning signs. Fortunately, these cases are pretty rare.

In an attempt to prevent stillbirth, your care provider may advise you to perform fetal kick counts (see page 30). The idea is that you might be able to feel decreased fetal movement and come in for evaluation and potentially be delivered before the stillbirth happens. There are many anecdotal cases of this being an effective way of preventing stillbirth. However, one recent study of more than 400,000 women who performed a very specific fetal kick protocol for detecting reduced fetal movements showed that even with a precisely defined protocol, the rate of stillbirth was not decreased. The good news in this study was that the rate of stillbirth was found to be very low: about four out of every 1,000 pregnancies whether kick counts were done or not. Some people may read this and feel frustrated or powerless because it appears that a pregnant person cannot realistically detect an impending stillbirth. Another, more positive way of looking at this is that it takes the responsibility for sudden stillbirth off the pregnant person's shoulders. When a tragedy like this happens, it is very common to start questioning what one might have done to cause the event or what one might have done differently to prevent the event. There may be a tremendous feeling of guilt in these situations. Talking to a counselor or therapist and finding a support group following a stillbirth are recommended. StillStanding-Mag.com is a good resource for support.

In some pregnancies, there may be warning signs that there is an increased risk of stillbirth, providing the potential to prevent these losses. These pregnancies are monitored with nonstress tests (see page 31) and in some cases with advanced ultrasound techniques. If the test results suggest a very high risk of stillbirth, then the baby might be delivered early. One example is when poor fetal growth is detected during prenatal care. Babies who are not growing well have a higher chance of stillbirth compared to babies who are growing at an expected rate, so this is a warning sign. Growth-restricted babies are monitored and delivered at 37 to 39 weeks, but in severe cases may be delivered sooner. Another condition that has been associated with an increased risk of stillbirth is cholestasis, which is characterized by intense total body itching without a rash. Recent guidelines have suggested that these babies should be delivered at 36 weeks, but delivery dates are adjusted based on assessed risk. Another situation in which stillbirth might be prevented is when preeclampsia develops. Pregnancies with preeclampsia are monitored very closely. If the condition appears mild, the goal is to get to 37 weeks and then deliver. If the preeclampsia progresses to a severe form, it is usually best to deliver the baby early. Ending the pregnancy at the right time in cases of preeclampsia can prevent some stillbirths.

Other potentially preventable causes of stillbirth include things like uncontrolled diabetes or certain recreational drugs (like cocaine or methamphetamines). Smoking is also associated with stillbirth. Keeping diabetes under good control and avoiding smoking and drug use will prevent some stillbirths.

The final point to mention is that there are a small number of stillbirths in the last weeks of pregnancy, after 39 weeks, even in uncomplicated pregnancies. Inducing labor once the pregnancy is full term or late term will prevent some of these rare stillbirths.

However, there are some downsides to induction of labor, and you may not wish to have your labor induced. This decision usually requires detailed conversations in the last weeks of pregnancy so that you can make an informed decision regarding whether you prefer to be induced or continue to wait for natural labor. (See page 185 for a discussion of post-term pregnancy.) Although this close fetal monitoring and strategically timed delivery will prevent some stillbirths, we cannot prevent *all* stillbirths because sometimes they happen suddenly without warning.

Q. What can I expect physically after a miscarriage?

Sometimes you discover you're miscarrying because you're having pain and bleeding. When evaluated it turns out you are in the process of a miscarriage. In other cases, an evaluation may reveal that the pregnancy is no longer developing but is still inside the uterus and there is no sign of miscarriage yet. There are a few choices in these situations. One is to let the miscarriage happen on its own. Another is to take medications that stimulate the miscarriage to occur. The third option is to have a D&C (dilation and curettage), which involves using medical instruments to physically remove the pregnancy from the uterus. This is often performed in an OR, although there may be some situations where it can be performed in an office-like setting.

During a spontaneous or medically induced first trimester miscarriage, you're likely to feel cramps, similar to or slightly worse than what you feel during your monthly periods. There will also be bleeding, and it is likely to be heavier than a period. You can also expect to see some blood clots. In an early miscarriage, you may not see an actual fetus if it is still very small. You may notice passage of a deflated sac-like structure, perhaps the size of a large grape or small plum. When the miscarriage is complete, the cramping will calm down and the bleeding will slow down to light bleeding or spotting. Some miscarriages will complete over the course of a few hours in one day, but usually they take a few days.

A miscarriage will complete itself without the need for any medical interventions about 80 percent of the time. Sometimes a D&C might be needed to complete the process. During a miscarriage, you don't need to go to the hospital if the bleeding is reasonable, the pain is tolerable, and you're feeling okay other than the cramping. If the bleeding gets so heavy that it scares you or if you begin to feel dizzy or light-headed, then you should call your care provider or go to the hospital. For pain you can take ibuprofen or Tylenol. If your pain becomes too severe or if you develop a fever, you should go to the hospital immediately.

After the miscarriage has completed, you may continue to have light spotting for a few days or even a week or two. If you have a history of regular monthly periods, you should expect to have your next period within one to two months. The urine pregnancy test will stay positive for a short time until your body eliminates the pregnancy hormone hCG from your system. Sometimes the first few cycles after a miscarriage can be irregular, but you should get back to your regular cycles within two or three months.

Q. When can I start trying to conceive again after a loss?

Studies have shown that there is no measurable benefit to delaying subsequent pregnancy after a first trimester pregnancy loss. If the next pregnancy happens within three months of the miscarriage, there does not appear to be an increased risk of pregnancy complications like repeat miscarriage or preterm birth. Therefore, if it is your desire to try again for another pregnancy, there is no reason to avoid trying right away.

For second trimester miscarriage, there are fewer studies available that address this question. One study found that delaying pregnancy by at least three months was associated with a reduced risk of repeat miscarriage. Although this recommendation is less certain, it may still be prudent to delay pregnancy by three to six months after a second trimester miscarriage. For a stillbirth, the optimal delay would depend on how many weeks along you were at the time that the loss occurred. If the stillbirth was diagnosed in the second trimester, then the advice would be the same as for a second trimester miscarriage (delay three to six months). If the stillbirth happened in the third trimester, there are many studies that show increased risk of pregnancy complications (especially preterm birth) if the next pregnancy happens in less than 18 months. Therefore, if your last pregnancy ended in a third trimester stillbirth, then the general recommendation is to delay the next pregnancy by 18 months. You may need this time to recover both physically and emotionally as well.

Q. What can I expect emotionally after a loss?

Pregnancy loss refers to the loss of an unborn baby, and the term encompasses all types of losses, including losses during pregnancy, elective termination, and loss during childbirth. Pregnancy loss is often unexpected and traumatic. The first three to six months after the loss of a pregnancy are often the most challenging. Emotions such as anger, sadness, denial, and guilt can be expected during and after a loss.

These feelings, while overwhelming, are normal and valid after such a traumatic event, even and especially if you never had the opportunity to meet your baby.

After a loss, a parent may believe it was their fault. *"If only I hadn't... I should have known better... What if..."* These are common refrains in a parent's mind. They may look everywhere for a cause and a possible answer. Trying to find the reason for the loss is normal. Even when a miscarriage happens early in a pregnancy, it is painful. Regardless of how far along you were in your pregnancy or what type of loss occurs, this is a substantial loss, and you are allowed a grieving process.

Q. My partner and I are grieving differently. How can we get through this together?

Pregnancy loss may bring about different feelings for different people. It is important to remember that no two people grieve in exactly the same way. Communicate with your partner and find a good time to discuss how you're both feeling. There is no right or wrong way to grieve, and each of us needs support in different ways. Talking about your loss can help you heal together. You may consider attending a local support group together or seeking couples counseling.

Q. What resources are available to support me after a loss?

You are not alone. There are many other people who have experienced the loss of a pregnancy. In fact, one in four pregnancies ends in loss. Pregnancy loss support groups and counseling with a mental health professional are excellent resources as you grieve. There are miscarriage, abortion, and loss doulas specializing in ways to support before, during, and after your loss. There are also books and websites around loss that can help; see the Pregnancy Loss Support section in the Resources on page 216.

Q. What can I do to move toward healing emotionally after a loss?

When you're ready to move toward healing, there are several things that can help you along your journey.

Allow yourself space and time to feel anger, sadness, and denial. You're allowed to feel all of these. Create space to cry, scream, write, or sit in silence. There is no right way to grieve and heal. Some people prefer to be alone, while others want to engage with people during this time. Do what feels right for you.

Listen to your body and mind. Pregnancy loss can have a significant impact on your body. You may experience bleeding, cramps, and fatigue during and after a loss; you also may begin to lactate. Speak with your medical provider about ways to navigate these symptoms. Your body will also undergo hormonal changes, which can have an effect on mood and emotions. After a loss, postpartum mood and anxiety disorders can happen (see page 139 for more). Take the time you need to work through all of the emotions you're experiencing. Reach out to a trained mental health professional to help you navigate these feelings.

Know that healing is not linear. Some days are going to be better than others. There will be times when you feel you're making progress and an unexpected experience sets you back. A friend or coworker who doesn't know about the loss asking how much longer until delivery, seeing pregnancy announcements or gender reveals on social media, or approaching dates of pregnancy milestones and your estimated due date may trigger anger or sadness. It may be helpful to take a break from social media, unsubscribe from certain websites, and avoid certain people and events. It may be difficult to be around expecting parents, babies, or small children during this time. It's okay set limits and boundaries for yourself.

Honor your loss. For some, it may be helpful to your healing journey to do something to honor the loss. You may consider holding a memorial service, purchasing a special candle that you light in memory of your baby, or planting a tree or placing a memorial bench near your home. As a part of coping, some parents find it helpful to memorialize the loss by naming the baby. While this is a personal decision, these actions can help give meaning to your grief.

Seek support. Losing a baby changes you. While the grief may never go away, it will become manageable over time. If you're not in therapy, it may be helpful to reach out to a trained mental health professional to develop tools to help you explore your feelings and build healthy coping skills as you heal. You may want to seek out an online or in-person support group. Being around others who have experienced similar loss can provide validation and hope.

Q. How can I best support my partner or a loved one through a pregnancy loss?

If someone you love has experienced a pregnancy loss, you play an important role in their healing. Remember, there is nothing you can say or do to take away the pain they're experiencing; just being there can provide comfort. Here are some suggestions for how you might help.

Acknowledge the loss. The first step is to recognize the loss. While it may be uncomfortable, reach out and let the grieving parents know that you're sorry for the loss. You may want to offer to bring food, run errands, or sit with them. If your loved one doesn't seem receptive, give them time and space, but don't give up; continue checking in and offering support.

Don't try to "fix" it. It's natural to want to offer solutions. There is nothing we can do to take away the hurt. Statements like "At least your baby is in a better place" or "You can try again soon," while well-meaning, are dismissive and do not address the intense pain the parent may be feeling.

Listen. After a loss, parents may want to talk about their feelings, physical symptoms, or the hopes and dreams they had for the child. When we see someone we love hurting, we want to make it better, but all they need right now is an empathetic ear. Saying things like "I am glad you told me" or "I am sorry you're hurting, and I don't know what to say. I am here for you" is enough.

MEDICATIONS CHART

Medication/ supplement name	Typical use	First trimester
Acetaminophen (Tylenol)	Pain and fever reliever	Safe
Albuterol (Ventolin, Proair)	Asthma relief	Safe
Atorvastatin (Lipitor)	High cholesterol	Not safe
Beclomethasone inhaler (Qvar)	Asthma relief	Safe
Bisacodyl suppositories (Dulcolax)	Constipation relief/laxative	Safe
Budesonide inhaler (Pulmicort)	Asthma relief	Safe
Budesonide nasal spray (Rhinocort)	Allergies	Safe
Citalopram/Escitalopram (Celexa/Lexapro)	Depression, anxiety	Safe
Dextromethorphan (Robitussin)	Cough suppressant	Safe
Diphenhydramine (Benadryl, Nytol)	Antihistamine (for allergies, nausea, itching, insomnia)	Safe
Docusate (Colace, Surfak)	stool softener	Safe

Second trimester	Third trimester	Breastfeeding
Safe	Safe	Safe
Safe	Safe	Safe
Ask your doctor	Ask your doctor	Not safe
Safe	Safe	Safe
Safe	Safe	Safe
Safe	Safe	Safe
Safe	Safe	Safe
Safe	Ask your doctor	Ask your doctor
Safe	Safe	Safe
Safe	Ask your doctor	Ask your doctor
Safe	Safe	Safe

Medication/ supplement name	Typical use	First trimester
Eszopiclone (Lunesta)	Insomnia	Ask your doctor
Famotidine (Pepcid)	Heartburn relief	Safe
Fluoxetine (Prozac)	Depression, anxiety, OCD, others	Safe
Fluticasone inhaler (Flovent)	Asthma relief	Safe
Fluticasone nasal spray (Flonase)	Allergy relief	Safe
Glipizide (Glucotrol)	Diabetes	Ask your doctor
Glyburide (Diabeta, Glynase)	Diabetes	Safe
Guaifenesin (Mucinex, Siltussin)	Expectorant (for loosening phlegm)	Safe
Hydrochlorothiazide (Microzide)	High blood pressure	Ask your doctor
Ibuprofen (Advil, Motrin)	Pain and fever reliever	Not safe
Insulin	Diabetes	Safe
Labetalol (Normodyne, Trandate)	High blood pressure	Safe
Levothyroxine (Synthroid, Levoxyl)	Hypothyroidism	Safe

Second trimester	Third trimester	Breastfeeding
Ask your doctor	Ask your doctor	Ask your doctor
Safe	Safe	Safe
Safe	Ask your doctor	Ask your doctor
Safe	Safe	Safe
Safe	Safe	Safe
Ask your doctor	Ask your doctor	Ask your doctor
Safe	Safe	Safe
Safe	Safe	Safe
Ask your doctor	Ask your doctor	Ask your doctor
Ask your doctor	Not safe	Safe
Safe	Safe	Safe
Safe	Safe	Safe
Safe	Safe	Safe

Medication/ supplement name	Typical use	First trimester
Lisinopril (Zestril, Qbrelis)	High blood pressure	Ask your doctor
Metformin (Glucophage)	Diabetes, polycystic ovary syndrome (PCOS)	Safe
Methimazole (Tapazole)	Hyperthyroidism	Ask your doctor
Methyldopa (Aldomet)	High blood pressure	Safe
Nifedipine (Procardia)	High blood pressure	Safe
Omeprazole (Prilosec, Zegerid)	Heartburn	Safe
Paroxetine (Paxil)	Depression, anxiety, OCD, PTSD, others	Ask your doctor
Propylthiouracil (PTU, Propycil)	Hyperthyroidism	Safe
Pseudoephedrine (Sudafed)	Nasal congestion	Not safe
Ranitidine (Zantac)	Heartburn	Ask your doctor
Sertraline (Zoloft)	Depression, OCD, PTSD, others	Safe
Zolpidem (ambien)	Insomnia	Ask your doctor

Second trimester	Third trimester	Breastfeeding
Not safe	Not safe	Ask your doctor
Safe	Safe	Safe
Safe	Safe	Safe
Safe	Safe	Safe
Safe	Safe	Safe
Safe	Safe	Safe
Safe	Ask your doctor	Safe
Ask your doctor	Ask your doctor	Ask your doctor
Ask your doctor	Ask your doctor	Not safe
Ask your doctor	Ask your doctor	Ask your doctor
Safe	Ask your doctor	Ask your doctor
Ask your doctor	Ask your doctor	Ask your doctor

GLOSSARY
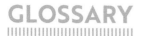

Amniocentesis. A procedure in which a needle is inserted into the uterine cavity under ultrasound guidance to collect a sample of amniotic fluid for genetic testing.

Amniotic fluid. The fluid that surrounds your baby in utero. It serves as a protective cushion for your baby and also contains important nutrients and antibodies. Your fluid levels will be monitored throughout pregnancy, and leaking fluid, also known as your water breaking, can be an indicator of labor starting.

Braxton-Hicks contractions. These are practice contractions and can last for several seconds or several minutes, but they do not hurt (although they can be uncomfortable) and should not occur in any sort of pattern. They typically start toward the end of your pregnancy, but if this isn't your first pregnancy, you may feel them as early as the second trimester.

Birth plan. A birth plan or list of birth preferences is a way for you to communicate your desires regarding labor, birth, and postpartum/newborn care with your care provider.

Breech position. Babies who are in a bottom-down (or feet-down) position.

Cervix dilation and effacement. Your cervix is the opening between your uterus and your vagina. During labor your cervix will dilate, or widen, and efface, or become thinner so it can stretch for your baby to pass through and be born. Many providers use the term "complete" to describe full dilation (10 centimeters dilated) and full effacement (100 percent effaced) and use these measurements as an indicator for when you're ready to push your baby out.

Cesarean birth. Also known as a cesarean section or C-section. This is a surgical birth where an incision is made in your lower abdomen and your baby is delivered by your doctor. Cesareans can typically be performed with the use of an epidural or spinal block; in this situation you won't feel the surgery but can remain awake during it. In some cases, general anesthesia is required.

Doula. A nonmedical professional who is trained in assisting birthing parents through pregnancy and postpartum. Their services may include prenatal education and advice, assistance in labor, assisting with feeding, baby care, and other postpartum care. Often, doulas will help you interact with other medical professionals to help ensure that your questions are being answered and that your needs are being met.

Ectopic pregnancy. When the embryo implants somewhere other than the uterus, e.g., within a fallopian tube. Symptoms include extreme abdominal pain and vaginal bleeding. It can cause your fallopian tube to burst open and requires immediate medical attention.

Epidural. A form of pain medication that is injected into a space around the nerves of your spinal cord on your lower back. It has the effect of providing pain relief from the waist down while allowing you to remain conscious for the birth of your baby.

Episiotomy. A surgical incision in the bottom of the vagina during childbirth to make the opening larger. The use of episiotomies in modern care should be limited to specific situations, such as emergencies where the baby needs to be delivered immediately.

Gestational diabetes. A type of diabetes that develops during pregnancy and causes high blood sugar that can affect your and your baby's health. You will be tested for GD between 24 and 28 weeks of pregnancy and will discuss your results and management with your care provider.

Group B strep (GBS) test. A test done on almost all pregnant people between 36 and 38 weeks to screen for the presence of group B streptococcus, one of the many bacteria that may be living in a healthy person's body under normal circumstances. However, it can be transmitted to the baby and make the baby very sick after birth in about 2 percent of cases, which is why this test is done.

Miscarriage. The term for the loss of a pregnancy prior to 20 weeks. After 20 weeks, a loss is called a stillbirth.

Obstetrics. This term refers to the specialty of caring for pregnant women during pregnancy and childbirth.

Operative vaginal delivery. This is a vaginal delivery where a medical instrument, either a vacuum or a pair of forceps, is used to help the baby be born.

Pelvic floor. This is the group of muscles and connective tissues that are underneath the pelvis. They support your bowels, vagina, uterus, and bladder.

Perinatal mood and anxiety disorders (PMADs). Mood disorders, including depression, anxiety, and psychosis, that occur during pregnancy or within one year after delivery due to the drastic shift in hormones and immense changes during pregnancy and postpartum.

Perinatologist. A doctor who specializes in the care of complicated pregnancies due to either a maternal health condition or a fetal health condition. Also known as a maternal-fetal medicine specialist.

Perineum. The space between your anus and vagina that stretches and often tears during childbirth. It is very stretchy tissue that typically heals quickly.

Physiological birth. This is a term used for labor and childbirth that progresses on its own accord without medical intervention.

Placenta accreta. When the placenta grows too deeply into the uterine wall, preventing it from detaching safely after birth. This is more common with pregnancies after a prior cesarean, as the placenta can grow into the scar tissues from a previous surgical birth.

Placenta previa. When the placenta attaches close to or over the cervix, preventing the baby from being born vaginally.

Preeclampsia. A serious condition involving high blood pressure that usually develops sometime after 20 weeks of pregnancy.

Symptoms include swelling, headaches, and blurriness of vision. Sometimes there are no symptoms at all, which is why your blood pressure and urine are tested at each prenatal appointment. The only way to treat preeclampsia is for your baby to be born.

Preterm labor. Labor that begins prior to 37 weeks of pregnancy.

Rupture of membranes. Also known as "water breaking," this is an indicator of the beginning of labor. Sometimes your water will break without contractions starting; this is known as premature rupture of membranes (PROM). Other times, your care provider will rupture your membranes as a form of induction or to augment your labor.

Ultrasound. An imaging method that uses high-frequency waves to produce images of structures within your body. Typically, three ultrasounds are performed in pregnancy. The first occurs when pregnancy is discovered to confirm the number of babies and gestational age. The second is the nuchal translucency ultrasound (between 11 weeks and 14 weeks and two days) to gauge if the baby is at increased risk for having an underlying chromosomal condition such as Down syndrome, another genetic condition, or a physical birth defect. The last one is the anatomy scan (between 18 and 22 weeks), a detailed examination of your baby to see if your baby is growing normally.

Vaginal birth after cesarean (VBAC). When you have had a cesarean section previously and are planning for a vaginal birth with your subsequent pregnancy.

RESOURCES
||||||||||||||||||||||||||||||||||||||

Pregnancy

Medications during pregnancy: MotherToBaby.org
Plus-size pregnancy: PlusSizeBirth.com and SizeFriendly.com
Twins and multiples: Twiniversity.com
Find a chiropractor: ICPA4Kids.com
Baby positioning: SpinningBabies.com
National Accreta Foundation: PreventAccreta.org

Birth

***The Birth Hour*'s "Know Your Options" online course:**
TheBirthHour.com
Listen to birth stories: TheBirthHour.com/birth-stories
Find a doula: DoulaMatch.net or DONA.org
Evidence Based Birth: EvidenceBasedBirth.com
Compare hospitals and view statistics: LeapfrogGroup.org or
BabyFriendlyUSA.org
International Cesarean Awareness Network: ICAN-Online.org
Vaginal birth after cesarean: VBACFacts.com
Vaginal breech delivery: InformedPregnancy.com/heads-up
Birthing Instincts with Dr. Stu: BirthingInstincts.com
Cord blood donation: BeTheMatch.org
Premature infants: MarchofDimes.org and GrahamsFoundation.org
Lamaze International: Lamaze.org
The Bradley Method: BradleyBirth.com
HypnoBirthing: US.HypnoBirthing.com
Birthing from Within: BirthingFromWithin.com
LGBTQ+-inclusive birthing resources: BirthForEverybody.org
Intersex resources: interACTadvocates.org

Preparing for Baby

Universal Baby Registry: Babylist.com
Infant CPR class: RedCross.org
Car seat installation: SafeKids.org or TheTotSquad.com

Breastfeeding Support

La Leche League International: LLLI.org
Help getting a breast pump through insurance: AeroflowBreast
Pumps.com
Find a lactation consultant: ILCA.org or USLCA.org
Evidence-based information on breastfeeding: KellyMom.com
The Birth Hour's "Back-2-Work Breastfeeding" online course:
TheBirthHour.com
The Birth Hour's "Quick Start Breastfeeding" download: TheBirth
Hour.com/breastfeeding
The Birth Hour's "Bottle Feeding" video: TheBirthHour.com/bottle

Newborn Care

Newborn sleep tips and online course: TakingCaraBabies.com
"Know Your Options" online course, newborn care module:
TheBirthHour.com
The Period of Purple Crying: PURPLECrying.info

Recommended books:
» *The Wonder Weeks: How to Stimulate Your Baby's Mental Development and Help Him Turn His 10 Predictable, Great, Fussy
  Phases into Magical Leaps Forward* by Frans X. Plooij and Hetty
  van de Rijt
» *The Happiest Baby on the Block: The New Way to Calm Crying
  and Help Your Newborn Baby Sleep Longer* by Dr. Harvey Karp
» *Cribsheet: A Data-Driven Guide to Better, More Relaxed Parenting, from Birth to Preschool* by Emily Oster

Postpartum Support and Recovery

Postpartum info: Postpartumprogress.com
Postpartum support 24/7 hotline: Postpartum.net
Diastatis recti and pelvic-floor recovery: MUTUsystem.com

Pregnancy Loss Support

Recommended books:

» *Empty Cradle, Broken Heart: Surviving the Death of Your Baby* by Deborah L. Davis

» *Grieving the Child I Never Knew: A Devotional Companion for Comfort in the Loss of Your Unborn or Newly Born Child* by Kathe Wunnenberg

» *Empty Arms: Coping after Miscarriage, Stillbirth, and Infant Death* by Sherokee Ilse

» *Surviving Miscarriage: You Are Not Alone* by Stacey McLaughlin, PhD

» *I Never Held You: Miscarriage, Grief, Healing, and Recovery* by Ellen DuBois and Dr. Linda Backman

Recommended websites:

M.E.N.D., Mend.org
Return to Zero: H.O.P.E., RtzHope.org
MISS Foundation, MISSFoundation.org
SHARE Pregnancy and Infant Loss Support, Nationalshare.org
Solace for Mothers (birth trauma recovery), SolaceforMothers.org
Star Legacy Foundation (support groups), StarLegacyFoundation.org/support-groups
Now I Lay Me Down to Sleep, NowILayMeDowntoSleep.org
Still Birth Day, StillBirthDay.com
Still Standing Magazine, StillStandingMag.com
Pregnancy After Loss Support (PALS), PregnancyAfterLossSupport.org
Instagram.com/ihadamiscarriage

Smartphone Apps

Ovia Parenting: To keep track of baby's daily schedule.

The Wonder Weeks: To note baby's developmental leaps.

Expectful: Pregnancy and postpartum guided meditations.

Breastfeeding Solutions: Help with common breastfeeding issues.

LactMed: A database of drugs and supplements that may have effects on a nursing baby and alternative options to consider.

REFERENCES
||||||||||||||||||||||||||||||||||||||||||

Alfirevic, Z., et al. "Continuous Cardiotocography (CTG) as a Form of Electronic Fetal Monitoring (EFM) for Fetal Assessment During Labour." *Cochrane Database of Systematic Reviews* 3 (July 2006): CD006066. doi:10.1002/14651858.CD006066.pub3.

American College of Obstetricians and Gynecologists. "Marijuana Use During Pregnancy and Lactation." Accessed November 26, 2019. https://www.acog.org/Clinical-Guidance-and-Publications/Committee -Opinions/Committee-on-Obstetric-Practice/Marijuana-Use-During -Pregnancy-and-Lactation.

American Congress of Obstetricians and Gynecologists. "Practice Bulletin no. 102: Management of Stillbirth." *Obstetrics and Gynecology* 113, no. 3 (March 2009): 748–61. doi:10.1097/AOG.0b013e31819e9ee2.

American Congress of Obstetricians and Gynecologists. "Practice Bulletin no. 145: Antepartum Fetal Surveillance." *Obstetrics and Gynecology* (July 2014). doi:10.1097/01.AOG.0000451759.90082.7b.

American Congress of Obstetricians and Gynecologists. "Practice Bulletin no. 146: Management of Late-Term and Postterm Pregnancies." *Obstetrics and Gynecology* 124, no. 2 part 1 (August 2014): 390–96. doi:10.1097/01.AOG.0000452744.06088.48.

American Congress of Obstetricians and Gynecologists. "Practice Bulletin no. 161: External Cephalic Version." *Obstetrics and Gynecology* 127, no. 2 (February 2016): e54–61. doi:10.1097/AOG.0000000000001312.

American Congress of Obstetricians and Gynecologists. "Practice Bulletin no. 171: Management of Preterm Labor." *Obstetrics and Gynecology* 128, no. 4 (October 2016): e155–64. doi:10.1097/ AOG.0000000000001711.

American Congress of Obstetricians and Gynecologists. "Practice Bulletin no. 173: Fetal Macrosomia." *Obstetrics and Gynecology* 28, no. 5 (November 2016): e195–209. doi:10.1097/AOG.0000000000001767.

American Psychiatric Association. *Diagnostic and Statistical Manual of Mental Disorders*, 5th ed. American Psychiatric Publishing, 2013.

Berghella, V., and A. D. Mackeen. "Cervical Length Screening with Ultrasound-Indicated Cerclage Compared with History-Indicated Cerclage for Prevention of Preterm Birth: A Meta-Analysis." *Obstetrics & Gynecology* (July 2011): 148–155. doi:10.1097/AOG.0b013e31821fd5b0.

Berhan, Y., and A. Haileamlak. "The Risks of Planned Vaginal Breech Delivery versus Planned Caesarean Section for Term Breech Birth: A Meta-Analysis Including Observational Studies." *BJOG* 123, no. 1 (January 2016): 49–57. doi:10.1111/1471-0528.13524.

Bigelow, C. A., and A. S. Bryant. "Short Interpregnancy Intervals: An Evidence-Based Guide for Clinicians." *Obstetrical & Gynecological Survey* 70, no. 7 (July 2015): 458–464. doi:10.1097/OGX.0000000000000195.

Black, M., et al. "Planned Cesarean Delivery at Term and Adverse Outcomes in Childhood Health." *JAMA* 314, no. 21 (December 2015): 2271–79. doi:10.1001/jama.2015.16176.

Blackwell, S. C., et al. "17-OHPC to Prevent Recurrent Preterm Birth in Singleton Gestations (PROLONG Study): A Multi-Center, International, Randomized Double-Blind Trial." *American Journal of Perinatology* (October 2019). doi:10.1055/s-0039-3400227.

Blix, E., et al. "Intermittent Auscultation Fetal Monitoring during Labour: A Systematic Scoping Review to Identify Methods, Effects, and Accuracy." *PLOS ONE* 14, no. 7 (July 2019): e0219573. doi:10.1371/journal.pone.0219573.

Boschert, Sherry. "Use 6-cm Dilation to Judge Labor Progress." *MDEdge ObGyn*. June 20, 2013. https://www.mdedge.com/obgyn/article/59333/womens-health/use-6-cm-dilation-judge-labor-progress.

Bower, K. M., et al. "Experiences of Racism and Preterm Birth: Findings from a Pregnancy Risk Assessment Monitoring System, 2004 through 2012," *Women's Health Issues* 28, no. 6 (November 2018): 495–501. doi:10.1016/j.whi.2018.06.002.

Cavallin, F., et al. "Delayed Cord Clamping versus Early Cord Clamping in Elective Cesarean Section: A Randomized Controlled Trial." *Neonatology* 116, no. 3 (2019): 252–59. doi:10.1159/000500325.

Centers for Disease Control and Prevention. "Cesarean Delivery Rate by State." Accessed November 25, 2019. https://www.cdc.gov/nchs/pressroom/sosmap/cesarean_births/cesareans.htm.

Centers for Disease Control and Prevention. "Depression among Women." Accessed October 3, 2019. https://www.cdc.gov/reproductivehealth/depression/index.htm.

Chen, C., et al. "Influences of Cesarean Delivery on Breastfeeding Practices and Duration: A Prospective Cohort Study." *Journal of Human Lactation* 34, no. 3 (January 2018): 526–34. doi:10.1177/0890334417741434.

Ciardulli, A., et al. "Less Restrictive Food Intake during Labor in Low-risk Singleton Pregnancies: A Systematic Review and Meta-Analysis." *Obstetrics and Gynecology* 129, no. 3 (March 2017): 473–80. doi:10.1097/AOG.0000000000001898.

Cox, J. L., et al. "Detection of Postnatal Depression: Development of the 10-Item Edinburgh Postnatal Depression Scale." *British Journal of Psychiatry* 150, no. 6 (June 1987): 782–86. doi:10.1192/bjp.150.6.782.

Durst, J. K., et al. "Resolution of a Low–Lying Placenta and Placenta Previa Diagnosed at the Midtrimester Anatomy Scan." *Journal of Ultrasound in Medicine* 37, no. 8 (August 2018): 2011–19. doi:10.1002/jum.14554.

Easter, S. R., J. N. Robinson, et al. "The U.S. Twin Delivery Volume and Association with Cesarean Delivery Rates: A Hospital-Level Analysis." *American Journal of Perinatology* 35, no. 4 (2018): 345–53. doi:10.1055/s-0037-1607316.

Evidence Based Birth. "Evidence on: Premature Rupture of Membranes." Accessed November 8, 2019. https://evidencebasedbirth.com/evidence-inducing-labor-water-breaks-term/.

Evidence Based Birth. "Natural Labor Induction Series: Evidence on Evening Primrose Oil." Accessed November 8, 2019. https://evidencebasedbirth.com/evidence-using-evening-primrose-oil-for-natural-labor-induction/.

Ghaedrahmati, M., et al. "Postpartum Depression Risk Factors: A Narrative Review." *Journal of Education and Health Promotion* 6, no. 60 (2017). doi:10.4103/jehp.jehp_9_16.

Ghaeri, Brian. "How to Choose Your Provider: Does Laser Vs Scissors Matter?" https://www.drghaheri.com/blog/2014/3/laser-vs-scissors-how-to-choose-your-provider.

Haas, D. M., et al. "Progestogen for Preventing Miscarriage in Women with Recurrent Miscarriage of Unclear Etiology." *Cochrane Database of Systematic Reviews* (October 2018): CD003511. doi:10.1002/14651858.CD003511.pub5.

Jain, V. "Choosing Wisely: Bedrest—A Panacea for All That Ails the Gravida?" *Journal of Obstetrics and Gynecology Canada* J41, no. 7 (July 2019): 971–73. doi:10.1016/j.jogc.2019.03.004.

Jansen, C. H. J. R., et al. "Vaginal Delivery in Women with a Low-Lying Placenta: A Systematic Review and Meta-Analysis." *BJOG* 126, no. 9 (August 2019): 1118–26. doi:10.1111/1471-0528.15622.

Kainu, J. P., E. Halmesmäki, et al. "Persistent Pain after Cesarean Delivery and Vaginal Delivery: A Prospective Cohort Study." *Anesthesia and Analgesia* 123, no. 6 (December 2016): 1535–45. doi:10.1213/ANE.0000000000001619.

Kangatharan, C., et al. "Interpregnancy Interval Following Miscarriage and Adverse Pregnancy Outcomes: Systematic Review and Meta-analysis." *Human Reproduction Update* 23, no. 2 (March 2017): 221–31. doi:10.1093/humupd/dmw043.

Kersting, Annette, and Brigitte Wagner. "Complicated Grief after Perinatal Loss." *Dialogues in Clinical Neuroscience* 14, no. 2 (June 2012): 187–94. Accessed December 28, 2019. https://www.ncbi.nlm.nih.gov/pmc/articles/PMC3384447/.

Lambert, N., et al. "Rubella." *Lancet* 385, no. 9984 (2016): 2297–307. doi:10.1016/S0140-6736(14)60539-0.

Levin, H. I., et al. "Activity Restriction and Risk of Preterm Delivery." *The Journal of Maternal-Fetal & Neonatal Medicine* 31, no. 16 (August 2018): 2136–40. doi:10.1080/14767058.2017.1337738.

Mangesi, L., et al. "Fetal Movement Counting for Assessment of Fetal Wellbeing." *Cochrane Database of Systematic Reviews* 10 (2015): CD004909. doi:10.1002/14651858.CD004909.pub3.

March of Dimes. "Caffeine in Pregnancy." Accessed November 10, 2019. https://www.marchofdimes.org/pregnancy/caffeine-in-pregnancy.aspx.

Matenchuk, Brittany, et al. "Prenatal Bedrest in Developed and Developing Regions: A Systematic Review and Meta-Analysis." *CMAJ Open* 7, no. 3 (July 2019): E435–45. doi:10.9778/cmajo.20190014.

Medela.com. "Why Is Colostrum So Important?" Accessed November 10, 2019. https://www.medela.com/breastfeeding/mums-journey/colostrum.

Nabhan, A. F., and Y. A. Abdelmoula. "Amniotic Fluid Index versus Single Deepest Vertical Pocket: A Meta-Analysis of Randomized Controlled Trials." *International Journal of Gynecology & Obstetrics* 104 (March 2009): 184–88. doi:10.1016/j.ijgo.2008.10.018.

Norman, J. E., et al. "Awareness of Fetal Movements and Care Package to Reduce Fetal Mortality (AFFIRM): A Stepped Wedge, Cluster-Randomized Trial." *Lancet* 392, no. 10158 (November 2018): 1629–38. doi:10.1016/S0140-6736(18)31543-5.

Okun, M.L., et al. "Changes in Sleep Quality, but Not Hormones Predict Time to Postpartum Depression Recurrence." *Journal of Affective Disorders* 130, no. 3 (May 2011): 378–84. doi:10.1016/j.jad.2010.07.015.

Purisch, S. E., et al. "Effect of Delayed versus Immediate Umbilical Cord Clamping on Maternal Blood Loss in Term Cesarean Delivery: A Randomized Clinical Trial." *JAMA* 322, no. 19 (November 2019): 1869–76. doi:10.1001/jama.2019.15995.

Rabie, N., et al. "Oligohydramnios in Complicated and Uncomplicated Pregnancy: A Systematic Review and Meta-Analysis. *Ultrasound in Obstetrics and Gynecology* 49, no. 4 (April 2017): 442–49. doi:10.1002/uog.15929.

Reitter, A., et al. "Mode of Birth in Twins: Data and Reflections." *Journal of Obstetrics and Gynecology* 38, no. 4 (May 2018): 502–10. doi:10.1080/01443615.2017.1393402.

Renfrew, M. J., et al. "Midwifery and Quality Care: Findings from a New Evidence-Informed Network for Maternal and Newborn Care." *Lancet* 384, no. 9948 (2015): 1129–45. doi:10.1016/S0140-6736(14)60789-3.

Roberge, S., et al. "Meta-Analysis on the Effect of Aspirin Use for Prevention of Preeclampsia on Placental Abruption and Antepartum Hemorrhage," *American Journal of Obstetrics & Gynecology* 218, no. 5 (May 2018): 483–89. doi:10.1016/j.ajog.2017.12.238.

Robert Peter, J., J. J. Ho, et al. "Symphysial Fundal Height (SFH) Measurement in Pregnancy for Detecting Abnormal Fetal Growth." *Cochrane Database of Systematic Reviews* 9 (2015): CD008136. doi:10.1002/14651858.CD008136.pub3.

Roberts, C. L., C. S. Algert, J. B. Ford, et al. "Association between Interpregnancy Interval and the Risk of Recurrent Loss after a Midtrimester Loss," *Human Reproduction* 31 (December 2016): 12, 2834–40. doi:10.1093/humrep/dew251.

Salomon, L. J., et al. "Risk of Miscarriage Following Amniocentesis or Chorionic Villus Sampling: Systematic Review of Literature and Updated Meta-Analysis." *Ultrasound in Obstetrics and Gynecology* 54, no. 4 (2019): 442–51. doi:10.1002/uog.20353.

Shi, Z., and A. MacBeth. "The Effectiveness of Mindfulness-Based Interventions on Maternal Perinatal Mental Health Outcomes: A Systematic Review." *Mindfulness* 8, no. 4 (2017): 823–47. doi:10.1007/s12671-016-0673-y.

Society for Maternal-Fetal Medicine. "What Is a Maternal-Fetal Medicine Subspecialist?" Accessed November 24, 2019. https://www.smfm.org/members/what-is-a-mfm.

Spong, C. Y., et al. "Preventing the First Cesarean Delivery: Summary of a Joint Eunice Kennedy Shriver National Institute of Child Health and Human Development, Society for Maternal-Fetal Medicine, and American College of Obstetricians and Gynecologists Workshop." *Obstetrics and Gynecology* 120, no. 5 (November 2012): 1181–93. doi: http://10.1097/AOG.0b013e3182704880.

Vedam, S., K. Stoll, et al. "Mapping Integration of Midwives across the United States: Impact on Access, Equity, and Outcomes." *PLoS ONE* 13, no. 2 (2018): e0192523. doi:10.1371/journal.pone.0192523.

Yip, B. H. K., et al. "Cesarean Section and Risk of Autism across Gestational Age: A Multi-National Cohort Study of 5 Million Births." *International Journal of Epidemiology* 46, no. 2 (April 2017): 429–39. doi:10.1093/ije/dyw336.

Young, Alison, and John Kelly. "Episiotomies Are Painful, Risky and Not Routinely Recommended. Dozens of Hospitals Are Doing Too Many." *USA Today*. May 21, 2019. https://www.usatoday.com/in-depth/news/investigations/deadly-deliveries/2019/05/21/episiotomy-vs-tearingmoms-cut-in-childbirth-despite-guidelines/3668035002/.

Zhu, Y., and C. Zhang. "Prevalence of Gestational Diabetes and Risk of Progression to Type 2 Diabetes: A Global Perspective." *Current Diabetes Reports* 16, no. 1 (January 2016): 7. doi:10.1007/s11892-015-0699-x.

Zlatnik, F. J. "Management of Premature Rupture of Membranes at Term." *Obstetrics and Gynecology Clinics of North America* 19, no. 2 (June 1992): 353–64. PMID: 1630743.

INDEX
||||||||||||||||||||||

ACKNOWLEDGMENTS

My heartfelt gratitude to the incredibly hardworking team at Callisto Media, most especially Ada Fung and Miranda Wicker, for helping this book come together.

Thank you to my co-authors Dr. Emiliano Chavira, MD, MPH, FACOG; Lindsey Meehleis, LM, CPM; and Courtney Butts, LMSW. I am so grateful for your expertise in writing this book and your passion for supporting families through pregnancy and new parenthood.

I am forever indebted to those who share their stories on *The Birth Hour* podcast and the listeners who receive them with open arms, free of judgment. Without your support, there would be no podcast, and there certainly would be no book.

To Adelaide, Darwin, and Harvey: Being pregnant with each of you taught me so much about myself and what my body is capable of, and your births showed me an inner strength I never could've imagined. And all of that was just the beginning—getting to see you grow up, explore the world, and discover your passions is the greatest gift. I'm so proud of each of you. Remember, kind and brave, my loves. Kind and brave.

Finally, thank you to Richard, my partner in life and parenthood— thank you for supporting all of my dreams and overcommitments. When I decided to write my second book in six months, your response was "How can I help?" and nothing but encouragement. The ways you lift me up in all that I do both professionally and as a mother are constant reminders that what we've built together is a beautiful partnership.

ABOUT THE AUTHOR

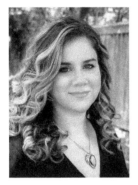

Bryn Huntpalmer is the founder of *The Birth Hour* podcast, which has been featured on the front page of Apple Podcasts and has more than 9 million downloads to date. She is passionate about helping people prepare for childbirth through the sharing of empowering and informative birth stories as well as an online, evidence-based childbirth course by *The Birth Hour*, called "Know Your Options."

This is Bryn's second book. Her first is a pregnancy and childbirth Amazon bestseller called *The First-Time Mom's Pregnancy Handbook: A Week-by-Week Guide from Conception through Baby's First 3 Months*.

Bryn lives in Austin, Texas, with her husband, Richard, and their three kids, Adelaide, Darwin, and Harvey. She considers it her most important job to raise her children to be kind, aware, and courageous human beings. Find Bryn at TheBirthHour.com or on social media: @thebirthhour or @brynessentials.